"A raw, honest and powerful book about the messy journey of healing after rape for the client and the impact that this has on her therapist too. *Both Sides of the Couch* is an important book that shines a light and offers hope."
MADELEINE BLACK, AUTHOR OF *UNBROKEN*

"Delicately written, with heartbreaking detail and searing honesty, *Both Sides of the Couch* is a hymn to the power of vulnerability."
ERIN KELLY, *SUNDAY TIMES* BESTSELLING AUTHOR

"As compulsively readable as a thriller but with the heart and depth of a modern classic in therapeutic writing. I will never forget this book."
SARAH HILARY, AWARD-WINNING AUTHOR

"What a powerful book. So insightful. So honest."
LOUISE BEECH, AUTHOR OF *EIGHTEEN SECONDS*

"Bold, courageous and compelling, this innovative dual-perspective account of recovery from trauma demonstrates how a therapeutic relationship built on compassion and trust can navigate the vicissitudes of therapy towards healing and hope. A hugely brave, honest and important piece of writing."

DR CHRIS MERRITT, CLINICAL PSYCHOLOGIST AND AUTHOR

Anna Wickins and
Paddy Magrane

BOTH SIDES OF THE COUCH

A story of recovery told by
a therapist and their client

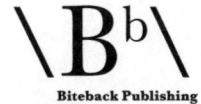

Biteback Publishing

First published in Great Britain in 2024 by
Biteback Publishing Ltd, London
Copyright © Anna Wickins and Paddy Magrane 2024

Anna Wickins and Paddy Magrane have asserted their rights under the Copyright,
Designs and Patents Act 1988 to be identified as the authors of this work.

All rights reserved. No part of this publication may be reproduced, stored in a retrieval system
or transmitted, in any form or by any means, without the publisher's prior permission in writing.

This book is sold subject to the condition that it shall not, by way of trade or otherwise,
be lent, resold, hired out or otherwise circulated without the publisher's prior consent in
any form of binding or cover other than that in which it is published and without a similar
condition, including this condition, being imposed on the subsequent purchaser.

Every reasonable effort has been made to trace copyright holders of material reproduced in
this book, but if any have been inadvertently overlooked the publisher would be glad to hear
from them.

ISBN 978-1-78590-892-7

10 9 8 7 6 5 4 3 2 1

A CIP catalogue record for this book is available from the British Library.

Set in FreightText Pro

Printed and bound in Great Britain by
CPI Group (UK) Ltd, Croydon CR0 4YY

ANNA

For Sam

PADDY

For Ella

*'The meeting of two personalities is like the contact of two
chemical substances: if there is any reaction,
both are transformed.'*
CARL JUNG

NOTE TO THE READER

Both Sides of the Couch is a therapeutic memoir about finding light in the darkest of places. For the authors, the path to recovery involved the examination and processing of historic trauma, much of which is described in the book. Readers should therefore be aware that the story discusses the impact of sexual violence, child sexual abuse and self-harm and contains a graphic depiction of self-harm.

The conversations in the book are based on Paddy's therapeutic case files and Anna's personal notes. They do not represent word-for-word transcripts but are retold to convey the essence of the exchanges.

The authors have changed some dates, names, identifying details and locations to maintain anonymity.

CHAPTER 1

Devon, July 2020

ANNA

I drive along the narrow country lanes towards our agreed meeting point, windows down, hair blowing wildly across my face. The hedgerows are filled with campion and cow parsley, and as I speed past, they blend into stripes of white and pink reminiscent of my daughter's favourite Drumstick sweets. It could be just another normal sunny day in Devon. It's almost too easy to forget where I'm going today.

I make a couple of left turns, and the early morning sun streams through the passenger side window. I catch sight of my bare arm as I change gear. The scars have almost faded beneath my tanned skin, but I know they're there. A constant reminder. A ball of dread begins to build in my stomach, twisting my insides, and a screaming voice in my head tells me not to go back to that place, to keep driving. I could go to the beach for the day, read a book under a tree, do *anything but this*. It's a strong temptation.

I pull in to the side of the road to let a tractor go by and it gives me a chance to pause. To breathe. Trying not to panic, I turn my attention back to the countryside and I hear a melodic sparrow's birdsong. At least I think it's a sparrow. Soft and sweet, yet it has a boldness. The more I focus on the sound, the more it soothes my nerves and increases my bravery. I can do this. I have to.

The farmer waves a 'thanks' as he passes. I wave back cheerfully, my panic contained for now.

I continue down the lane, swerving potholes, and park awkwardly. Paddy is already there in his car, waiting. He waves. For the second time today, I wave cheerfully but fraudulently back.

Hopping into his car, I ask him how he is before he can ask me the same question.

'Fine,' he replies.

I resist the temptation to mention that 'fine' isn't an answer, as he has so often pointed out to me.

'And you?'

'I'm OK,' I reply, sounding more optimistic than I am.

We can both feel the nerves, the anticipation, the sense of the unknown in the day ahead of us. There's an incongruence between what we're saying and how we're feeling, and we both know it. I'm certain that neither of us is feeling 'fine' or 'OK'.

It's a beautiful summer's day in 2020 and the public are

allowed to travel again after Covid restrictions have eased. While others are using their new-found freedom to visit loved ones, take much-needed holidays or explore new places, Paddy and I are travelling for a very different and unique reason.

I take a look around his immaculate car. It's a complete contrast to mine, which is littered with children's toys and crumbs.

'I've sanitised the entire car and I have plenty of hand gel,' he says. 'There are also masks and gloves in the boot.'

'Imagine how dodgy that would've sounded pre-Covid. Do you have a rope and shovel too?' I joke.

He laughs and I feel myself relax a little as I sink into the passenger seat. I'm ready.

———————————— " " ————————————

PADDY

'Seen anything good on Netflix?' I ask, accelerating onto the motorway.

As opening lines go, it's on a par with a hairdresser's 'Been anywhere nice recently?'

But there's a reason I've opted for something anodyne.

Anna and I have been working together for over two years by this point. It's not the longest I've seen a client, but the nature of our therapeutic relationship means that she knows me better than anyone else I've worked with.

Over the course of our sessions, I've revealed a number of aspects – both personal and mundane – of my life. Anna knows about my childhood and my experience of parenting. My life outside the therapy room.

The American psychotherapist Irvin Yalom likens self-disclosure to a kickstart. This is exactly how I experience it. Anna was often more inclined to open up if she'd heard me do the same. If I was prepared to be vulnerable, then she was too.

Self-disclosure served another purpose in our work. Sometimes, towards the end of a particularly difficult session, Anna needed a little help decompressing, so that she could leave therapy and face the journey home in a calm and grounded state. In those moments, we'd slip into a more conversational space, exchanging thoughts about the books and films we'd recently enjoyed.

Now, we're on our way to Bristol and face hours in the car together. We've agreed not to treat the entire trip as a therapy session. There is plenty of time for that once we reach our destination.

We talk about *Russian Doll*, a Netflix show we've both enjoyed about a woman who's trapped in a time loop, dying repeatedly only to return to a New York apartment where her birthday is being celebrated. There's something about the show that resonates with us both. Neither of us says it out loud, but I can't help wondering whether it's the protagonist, who is forever trying to figure out what's happened to her.

Our conversation fills the car, pushing other thoughts

out of my head. We've prepared so well for this moment. Drawing on her organisational skills and motivated by an understandable desire to retain a degree of control, Anna has compiled comprehensive risk assessments that consider every possible outcome of the trip. She is clutching several printouts filled with possible scenarios – panic attacks, nausea, dissociation – and how to manage them. I've discussed the trip at length with my supervisor, Sue, a therapist I see every month to discuss my client work. We're as ready as we could possibly be.

But this is still unknown territory. Few therapists attempt journeys like this: a visit to the scene of a client's trauma. It's sometimes incorporated into trauma-focused cognitive behavioural therapy (CBT), but it doesn't feature regularly in other therapeutic schools of thought. Our trip is unorthodox, to say the least.

I'm acutely aware we're out in the open, away from the safety and confinement of the counselling room. We're heading to a place filled with dark memories, where we'll inevitably collide with life, with all the unpredictable sights and sounds of a city – people chatting and arguing, distant sirens, music booming from cars. To complicate matters further, the country is only just emerging from lockdown, like an animal blinking hesitantly in the sunshine after months hibernating underground. The air is heavy with palpable uncertainty and anxiety.

The negative thoughts creep into my mind, spreading like ivy. I focus on the road, on staying in the conversation.

We've tried so many different tactics and strategies in our therapy sessions. This trip feels like the last throw of the dice. But Anna has worked so hard. She deserves to heal. We have to make this work.

CHAPTER 2

'All sorrows can be borne if you put them into a story or tell a story about them. But if we cannot find a way of telling our story, our story tells us – we dream these stories, we develop symptoms, or we find ourselves acting in ways we don't understand.'
STEPHEN GROSZ, THE EXAMINED LIFE:
HOW WE LOSE AND FIND OURSELVES

Devon, July 2018

ANNA

Two years previously, I found myself at the beginning of a very different journey.

I was sitting in the front of our family car – my husband Sam at the wheel and our three small children strapped securely into their car seats, each clutching a favourite teddy – with a bowl balanced on my lap.

I'd already thrown up twice before we left and although I had nothing left in my stomach, I wasn't confident that I'd manage the whole journey without needing to be sick again.

My suspicions were confirmed. Five minutes from our destination, we were forced to stop at the nearest coffee shop where I had my final nervous vomit.

I popped some chewing gum in my mouth and walked slowly across the cafe's car park. As I reached our car, I paused, my hand on the door. I didn't have to do this. We could drive away and have a family day out. Then, I looked at my children, innocence splashed across their faces, and reminded myself exactly why I was doing this. *Get a grip*, I thought.

A few minutes later, Sam dropped me at a house opposite a graveyard in an isolated, rural village – not the most auspicious location for a first therapy session. Our small children giggling and singing in the back of our car had helped to distract me from my nerves on the final leg of our journey, but now the time had come to get out and do this alone. I couldn't hide any longer. I had to face my fears.

I opened the car door to a blast of unbearable heat. We'd spent the past few days camping as a family and the lack of sleep, combined with the relentless scorching sun, had left us all feeling somewhat irritable. Anxiety about the impending appointment had heightened each day of the holiday and we had cut it short, returning a day early. Having spent the week in shorts and T-shirts, I'd panicked all morning about what to wear. I wanted to look professional, make a good impression. In the end, Sam thankfully took the decision out of my hands and pointed to a floor-length sundress. Always ready, I paired it with trainers, just in case I needed to run.

Head down, in case anyone saw me, I plodded up the driveway. My shame weighed me down heavily into the gravel. I approached the porch, scattered with honeysuckle, and by chance I looked down. I stopped abruptly, with my foot hovering over a majestic hornet. Berating myself for almost killing an innocent creature, I watched in awe as the bewitching insect flew busily between the sweet-smelling blooms, seemingly oblivious to its near-death experience.

I took a deep breath and tentatively pressed the doorbell, only to be greeted by a beautiful fox-red Labrador barking protectively through the door.

No one came.

I knocked a little too forcefully. The doorbell might be broken, but just in case I'd already annoyed the therapist, I took a few steps back. Still no answer. My nerves began to re-assert themselves and I started to feel like an inconvenience: a familiar sensation.

Perhaps I'd got the time wrong. Part of me hoped I had, and part of me hoped he wouldn't turn up at all.

I looked around to discover the hornet was no longer visible, its hypnotic buzz now silent. Suddenly, there was a razor-sharp pain on my shoulder and I watched as the large wasp flew away. Its yellow and black stripes, alluring only moments before, were now obviously hazardous. There was searing white-hot pain as the venom fired into my bloodstream.

I felt a stab of anger at the creature whose life I'd spared. Typical, I thought, that the things I'm most kind towards end up hurting me the most. I had started to regret this.

I retrieved my phone from my bag. We'd only had email contact before today and in my increasing panic, I'd forgotten we were complete strangers. I called the therapist's number.

'I think I'm outside your house,' I blurted out with no 'Hello' or introduction to who I was.

'Anna?' he replied. 'I'm so sorry, I'm running late. I'm stuck in traffic, but I'll be there soon.'

Not too soon, I hoped.

I spotted a bench near the front door and sat down to Google hornets, discovering that only the females sting. Adaptable and warrior-like, they can be vicious when their homes are threatened. It wasn't hard to relate to those qualities.

I'd give the therapy process six weeks. I would tell the therapist the bare minimum and he would fix me. *Six weeks*. It sounded like such a long time, a whole school summer holiday, but I believed that I owed it to Sam and to our children to be 'better'.

As I sat alone on the bench, hot and uncomfortable, I started to dread having to tell him the real reason I was there. It was a secret I'd hidden for nearly twenty years that had become increasingly difficult to ignore, bursting out in many unhelpful ways.

Would I have to tell him? If he *made* me tell him, then I'd do it in a matter-of-fact way, so he'd know it didn't bother me. That it was just an event in the past and I was strong enough not to let it affect me. I didn't want him to think I was weak or that I couldn't cope. I was already so embarrassed and ashamed to be there, to be asking for help, and ashamed of just being me.

———————————— " " ————————————

PADDY

When a new client starts therapy, I'm aware they're taking a big step, choosing to entrust their innermost thoughts and feelings to a stranger. That takes enormous courage.

I feel a sense of great responsibility. I want to prepare the ground for that first encounter, ensure the counselling room is calm and ordered and that my mind is emptied of external stresses, ready for whatever clients bring.

On the day of Anna's first session, I was far from prepared or stress-free. The whole week had been thrown into turmoil by the unexpected closure of my youngest daughter's specialist dyslexia school. My wife and I had fought hard to secure her a place, but now, just months into her time there, the school had suddenly closed its doors. Since then, we'd been travelling all over the West Country, desperate to find an alternative in time for September. But that day I'd mistimed the journey and got stuck in traffic on the way home.

Some ten minutes after the session was due to start, I tore up the drive, my shirt damp and clinging to me with sweat.

Anna was sitting on a bench outside the front door. She looked calm. My dog Lola was barking ferociously behind the front door. Hardly a warm welcome.

Normally, clients enter the house via a side door. It's to ensure that my work and my home are kept separate. I also think it's important to steer clients clear of the private spaces within, in case they start to construct a fantasy in their head of who I am. It's not that I wish to offer a completely blank canvas, but a client who sees a room filled with personal effects can unconsciously begin to draw conclusions, which can then influence how they interact with me and with therapy. Think, for example, how a photo of a therapist's child might affect a client struggling with infertility or someone who's divorced and alone, isolated from their family.

'You found me,' I said, attempting to sound calm and welcoming while my heart was hammering in my chest. 'I'm sorry I kept you waiting.'

'It's OK,' said Anna. 'Although I think I've been stung by a hornet.'

'Are you sure you want to continue with the session?'

Anna nodded.

Another client in the same pain might have elected to go home. In hindsight, Anna's decision was telling. As it turned out, she could withstand unbearable pain.

I unlocked the door, introducing Lola, whose barking ceased as soon as Anna stroked her. I led us through the sitting room, all but tripping over a vacuum cleaner. It felt like the session was descending into chaos with every step.

I told Anna I had an analgesic spray that would numb the pain and nipped upstairs to the bathroom to fetch it. Once I was back in the counselling room, I stood behind her and sprayed it directly onto the sting on her shoulder.

So here I was, a therapist who'd turned up late and stressed for his client's first session, who'd led her through his messy home rather than through the calm and contained side entrance and who was now invading her personal space. As the session unfurled, my actions assumed even more significance. Given what she described, it struck me that the last thing Anna needed was a strange man positioning himself directly behind her.

Finally, we settled.

'The sessions are fifty minutes long,' I hurriedly explained, keen not to waste any more of her time. 'And with the exception of my supervision and in the event that you were in danger of hurting yourself or someone else, the sessions are completely confidential.'

Anna was silent, squirming on the sofa.

'So,' I said, 'what has brought you to counselling?'

———————————— " " ————————————

ANNA

My leg began to shake and a wave of nausea hit me. Now I was going to have to talk.

My eyes dropped to the therapist's white Converse and my

lip started to tremble. 'I had a nightmare...' I whispered, as though someone had suddenly stolen my voice. I was unable to finish the sentence, as memories of the bad dream entered my head and the tears began to flow. I'd never cried in front of a stranger in my life and I felt embarrassed, almost penitent, believing that he must have thought I was highly unprofessional.

My mind wandered back to a few nights ago, to a terrifying nightmare that resulted in my first-ever panic attack.

I had woken suddenly, sitting up abruptly in bed with an audible gasp. Drenched in sweat and disorientated, I stumbled clumsily across the landing to the bathroom, the children's nightlights helping to guide my path. Barely making the toilet bowl, I vomited as quietly as I could, trying not to wake the peaceful house.

After emptying the contents of my stomach, I began to silently cry. The tears fell by themselves and splashed gently onto the floor, before they turned into sobs and I was gasping for breath. I lay down on the cool tiles as I felt invisible hands around my throat, squeezing every last breath out of me. I couldn't swallow and I couldn't remember how to breathe. The more I attempted to gulp air into my lungs, the more my chest and throat restricted. I was scared. Terrified, in fact. My thoughts were a confused muddle. Was I dying? Having anaphylaxis? My heartbeat was so deafening I was sure the rest of the house could hear it.

Eventually, my breathing became staccato and my heart rate slowed slightly. I willed myself to move. I heard my two-year-old turn over in his bed and my maternal instincts jolted me back into reality.

After making sure that everyone was safe and triple-checking that the front door was locked, I climbed back into bed, trying not to wake a soundly sleeping Sam. The sheets had cooled and dried from my sweaty nightmare and I started to shiver. As I lay wide awake, images and scenes from the dream began to play over and over again on a continuous loop. Spinning trees, a screeching car, a front door, blurred faces, smells and noises. I began to cry again, silently sobbing into the pillow until exhaustion took over and I fell into a restless sleep.

I don't know how long I'd been reliving that moment in front of Paddy – only a few seconds perhaps – but it was long enough to experience some of the sensations from the panic attack that had followed my nightmare. My breath had quickened and as I looked down at my wrist, my sports watch was flashing like I was sprinting, with my heartbeat at its peak. If only Paddy could just have read my mind, instead of me having to voice anything.

'Would you like to tell me about the nightmare?' Paddy gently asked.

His kindness was unsettling and yet reassuring and calming at the same time. I tried to ignore the instincts that were screaming at me to keep my mouth shut. Every time I'd tried to speak up in the past, it had backfired, badly.

Chewing the inside of my cheek, I shook my head and glanced longingly at the door. The exit. The escape route.

I was so tempted to run away and not come back. But as I was in the middle of nowhere and Sam wasn't coming to get me until the end of the session, I didn't have much choice. I reminded myself I was there for a reason and tried to be brave. I thought of the hornet's warrior-like spirit. I knew that I wasn't going to get anywhere unless I talked. My eyes rested on a map of Devon on the wall. It soothed me slightly. Maps have always brought me comfort and a sense of order and logic when I have felt lost or unsure.

'Yes... but not yet,' I managed to say.

Silence fell between us. His constant eye contact was unbearable. Fifty minutes felt like an eternity. I fidgeted under his gaze.

Unable to stand the awkward silence, I pulled out my phone.

'I've written some stuff down,' I said. 'It was actually quite cathartic.'

I hoped he would think that I had processed it all and was fine now. That I wasn't damaged or broken, and maybe I wouldn't have to come back again.

I unlocked my phone and froze as I stared at the screen. I was paralysed with indecision. There was more silence. I couldn't move, I couldn't talk. I didn't know what to do. I'd spent decades suppressing a secret and not wanting anyone to know, and yet I desperately needed to tell someone. I couldn't imagine or dare to hope what it might be like not to have to carry the sheer weight of my secrets. Maybe it would be OK if I wasn't planning to come back. I could let him read my notes and that would help me somehow. The nightmares would magically stop and I'd never have to see him again.

I passed him the phone, my hand shaking with nerves.

'Would you like me to read the notes?' he asked.

I hesitated. And while all of my instincts screamed NO, I nodded.

'To myself or out loud?'

'Out loud is fine,' I said. Although as soon as the words left my mouth, I regretted them.

―――――――――――――― " " ――――――――――――――

PADDY

As I read the words, it became clear that this was an account of an event that had occurred almost twenty years previously, while Anna was studying at university.

Although brief and unemotional, like an office memo, it was charged with electricity and filled with pain.

CHAPTER 3

Eighteen. Just started university. Flatmate's birthday. Drank a lot in our halls then went to a club. Was wearing clothes I wouldn't normally wear – borrowed from flatmates. Short skirt, vest and boots.

Got upset and ran out of the club without keys or coat.

Bumped into X not far from the club and cried. We were by a grassy area with trees and bushes and he took me behind a bush and we sat down. We kissed and then I stood up and said I needed to go home. He pushed me down...

Afterwards I ran back to my halls and saw friends. Was upset. Eventually one asked if I'd been... and I nodded.

Next day no one spoke to me. My friends wouldn't talk to me and eventually started sending me messages saying I was a slag and a liar etc.

Hung out with new friends and spent as little time as possible at my halls. Got on with life.

Last day before I went home for the summer. Alone in my flat. Didn't check the peephole. X came in and... Second time.

CHAPTER 4

Bristol, July 2020

ANNA

As we enter the city centre, it's eerily quiet. I mirror the silence and stop making conversation. I can't think of anything to say anyway.

Although I haven't been here for almost twenty years, I begin to recognise roads and landmarks and as we drive past grand civic buildings, I can feel my nerves build to an unbearable pitch. We stop briefly at a junction and I focus on the tick-tock of the car's indicator. It reminds me of a rollercoaster. The clack-clack-clack of the chain pulling the carriages up the first ascent, the fear building; except someone has forgotten to pull down the safety bar.

A wave of nausea hits me and I clench my teeth. I fidget and shift in my seat.

'You OK?' Paddy asks.

We're at the top hat, the highest point of the rollercoaster; the point of no return. I want to get off and retreat to safety. I realise I'm holding my breath and my knee is bouncing rapidly up and down. I don't want to shut him out; I need to make the most of this trip.

'I'm nervous,' I force myself to reply. And as I exhale, I can feel myself grow a little calmer – the pressure dissipating like dandelion seeds scattering through the breeze. Even after two years of therapy, I'm still surprised at the power of actually verbalising and acknowledging my emotions. The rollercoaster's safety bar is finally secured.

'Me too,' he confesses.

I know that the only way I'm getting off this rollercoaster is if I ride it to the end. With Paddy's admission that he's nervous too, it feels like he's joined me on the ride, although I'm still not looking forward to it.

Paddy parks and we both hesitantly get out of the car.

'Ready when you are,' he says.

I take a deep breath. I feel prepared and brave. I also feel scared and weak. This trip could reawaken all of my deepest fears or it could free me from the past. I want nothing more than to move on with my life. The trip is a risk we're both willing to take.

I pull my rucksack onto my shoulders, which are already tense with nerves, and start to walk. In my head, I have an order of the places I need to visit, which strangely has become the opposite of what I meticulously planned in the many months leading up to this moment. I think I'm saving the hardest parts for later.

'There's the museum and the uni buildings.' I'm pointing out the bloody obvious like a terrible tour guide. I know that I'm deflecting from what's going on inside me. Trying to hide the rising dread. But I'm scared that if I pay even the slightest bit of attention to it, the terror will overwhelm me and I won't be able to continue.

Fear has held me captive for the majority of the past twenty years. Today, I have the opportunity to confront it.

CHAPTER 5

'When we face pain in relationships our first response is often to sever bonds rather than to maintain commitment.'
BELL HOOKS, *ALL ABOUT LOVE: NEW VISIONS*

Devon, July 2018

ANNA

Despite Paddy reading softly and without emotion, his voice sounded like a scream. It hung in the air and I imagined myself grabbing handfuls of the words and shoving them back into the phone. It was too late – everything that I'd kept inside for so long was suddenly out.

As he finished reading, I realised that I'd teared up. I swiped at my eyes with a finger before he could see. It was a lot to share in one go. Especially with a stranger, even as kind as he was. I didn't deserve kindness.

Paddy handed me back the phone.

He said nothing.

I said nothing.

It was another excruciating silence. Why wasn't he saying anything? Was I in trouble?

———————————— " " ————————————

PADDY

Rushing to speak when Anna was silent seemed the wrong reaction, so I responded with a silence of my own. But I wanted to communicate an important message within it. Anna had just told me something that she'd held inside for nearly two decades. I wanted my silence, above all, to communicate acceptance.

When I eventually spoke, I was careful not to use the word 'rape'. For whatever reason (and it later became clear), she had chosen not to use it herself and it was critical that I remained within her frame of reference. I needed to hear what was being communicated and respond in a way that showed her I understood her inner world and what it meant to be her.

———————————— " " ————————————

ANNA

'Which part upset you?' he said, finally piercing the silence.

I was irritated that I hadn't hidden my tears well and that

he'd noticed. 'I don't want people to look at me differently,' I heard myself say.

With the exception of Sam, the people I'd told before had. I was certain of it. And at that moment, I was certain that Paddy thought less of me. Why wouldn't he? And why would he believe me when others hadn't?

'Did you report it?'

My shoulders dropped and I let out a disappointed sigh. That familiar and predictable question. I didn't report it, so I'm not a proper 'victim'.

I shook my head. *He doesn't believe me.*

I glanced up at him. His brow furrowed as he seemed to be searching for something to say. Another silence.

'You're not to blame, Anna.'

Fresh tears rapidly replaced the ones I'd wiped away. Tears of shame, embarrassment and mortification but also of relief and confusion at his kindness. Paddy wasn't saying he didn't believe me. He looked pointedly at the tissues next to me, but not wanting to make a fuss or admit I was upset, I used the back of my hand.

His empathy was frightening and I panicked – realising that I had let my defences down. My heart began to race and a sense of dread spread through my chest. It was frightening because I knew deep down it meant that he could see through the façade that I'd carefully constructed. The sturdy walls I'd built to protect myself from pain and rejection had suddenly crumbled, leaving me unguarded and exposed. A stupid mistake; I should have known better. I berated myself for showing weakness, for letting him see my tears. I was undeserving of any kindness. He had no idea! Of course I was to blame. Did he not read it properly? My defences came back up and I deeply regretted sharing my words with him.

'How does it feel, letting me read those words?' Paddy asked.

Fucking awful. Crushing. Like I've been promised a puppy and instead been shot at close range.

I composed myself. Sat a little taller.

'Good,' I replied, attempting a smile.

I didn't know why I had said it, but I knew that pleasing people was usually a good option. Safer, even.

———————————— " " ————————————

PADDY

All therapists make mistakes. I rarely hit on the perfect analogy, phrase or interpretation – the one that 'fits' the client, that makes them feel heard and understood at the deepest level – first time around. But with luck, those ill-fitting words act like stepping stones, helping therapist and client to move forwards together towards an understanding that does fit.

Inevitably, there are occasions when a mistake feels less constructive and more clumsy or insensitive. Asking Anna whether she'd reported the rapes struck me, almost immediately, as a misjudged comment. It placed responsibility on her, when she bore none. Why had I said it? The truth is I was reeling from the impact of her revelation – feeling, quite suddenly, out of my depth. I'd been practising for over ten years and in all that time had never encountered a client who'd been raped. In trying to lock on to facts, I'd hoped to gain some scaffolding. What I should have done was stay with her, precisely where she was.

'I'm glad I've found a counsellor,' I remember her saying towards the end of the session. 'I won't have to tell my story ever again.'

I doubted that would be the case. But there seemed little point drawing her attention to what lay ahead if she committed to the work. Hope is fundamental to therapeutic success.

As we drew to a close, I invited her to think about writing down the nightmare if she had it again. It might have seemed familiar to her, but the content could have useful things to impart, while possibly offering another route into the therapeutic work.

———————— " " ————————

ANNA

I felt extreme relief hearing our family car pull into the drive. The hour had been so painful and not only because of the hornet sting. In fact, in a strange way, that physical pain had provided a welcome distraction from the emotional pain I was trying so hard to avoid. I couldn't wait to leave and before I'd even walked out of the door, I knew I wasn't going to return.

CHAPTER 6

PADDY

Anna was at the beginning of a journey. Years before, I'd begun one of my own.

I was twenty-four years old when I first saw a therapist. I was an artist at the time, living in a rented basement flat with my girlfriend in north London. Every day, I cycled across the river to a studio in Bermondsey, where I shared a building with dozens of fellow painters and sculptors. The lack of common areas meant we spent our days isolated from each other, hunkered away in cold, damp rooms with tall ceilings and windows that offered bleak views of the rooftops of a grim, post-industrial corner of London. I'd been awarded a first at art college and left full of excitement and confidence about my future as a professional artist. But five years on, reality was biting. I tried to stage a show once a year, but even if I managed to sell a handful of paintings, it was never enough to live on. To boost my income, I signed on at the local job centre in Hackney, where I queued every fortnight with agitated, edgy claimants whose angry altercations with the staff frequently punctuated the tense, sour air.

Depression can hit suddenly, like a chill in the air when the winter sun disappears behind a cloud. Or it can creep over you slowly, like sea mist, until it coats your skin and clothes. This was how I experienced it. It was February, my breath turning to vapour in the studio, when I realised I had to seek help. A painting – a cold minimalist work which looked as lifeless as I felt – hung on the wall. I'd barely made a mark for weeks.

Like so many first-time clients, I had little idea where to find support. We had a dog-eared copy of the Yellow Pages in the flat (this was the early '90s, pre-internet) and one afternoon I scanned through the listings, feeling increasingly muddled and overwhelmed. There were hundreds of therapists listed: counsellors, psychiatrists, psychotherapists, psychologists, each name followed by a set of letters indicating their qualifications and the therapeutic models they offered. It was like attempting to read impenetrable coding. I was on the verge of giving up when a friend from art school, someone who'd confided in me about how she'd suffered with depression, recommended a Jungian psychoanalyst called Philip in Hampstead.

Looking back, I'm not sure I even researched what the Jungian approach entailed. I simply took the plunge. I knew that otherwise I'd procrastinate indefinitely.

As I climbed Haverstock Hill from the Tube station, my heart pounded in my chest – and not just from the exertion.

I'd rehearsed what I was going to say, but the more I walked, the more the nerves ate away at me, throwing obstacles in my path. What was I doing here? Was I really depressed? Was my issue worthy of therapeutic attention? I was still a product of my upbringing – father in the army, a private education – and while I'd learned to express myself at art school, feelings were another language altogether.

On the ground floor of the building in which Philip practised, there was an employment agency. Eyes rose from desks to watch me pass in the hallway. Another nutter visiting the shrink on the fifth floor, I imagined them thinking.

Philip greeted me at the open door. He was tall and bald, the beard that lined his jaw giving him the look of an Amish farmer. It was early evening and the warm, slightly stale air in the room suggested that he'd been seeing clients all day, their problems still lingering like dust motes. He invited me to sit in an armchair. My eyes scanned the room, taking in a number of softly ticking antique clocks, small wooden tribal figures, prints of Cézanne paintings and bookshelves groaning with large leather-bound volumes of Jungian and Freudian texts. In the very first minute, I formed the impression that I was in the presence of an intellectual superior, a view I never managed to shake.

The chairs in his room were arranged side by side but at slight angles, so I was aware of him but not looking directly at him.

And so began my analysis, a process that was to last four years.

I had so little understanding of what to expect that it took a while to understand how Philip operated, but the signs were there from the start.

'What's brought you here?' he asked, after he'd taken some details.

'I feel unproductive. Stuck.'

Silence.

It became so uncomfortable that I forced more words out of my mouth, attempting to qualify what I meant, to inject more meaning.

'I feel low. Depressed. Although that sounds a bit dramatic,' I added, trying to retract that last word. I'd hardly said anything, but already it felt like too much.

Silence was one of Philip's tools. Along with an aloof, mirror-like presence.

'Do you like Cézanne?' I remember asking once, hoping we could talk about the art on his walls for a change.

'I'm wondering why you feel it's important to ask that,' he replied.

Analysis transformed me in so many positive ways. My initial issue – the combination of depression, stagnation and paralysis – was merely the top layer. Underneath, with his help, I discovered more, much of which centred on the effect boarding school had had on me. Years later, this experience led me to study psychotherapy at the University of East London.

But by then, I knew I wanted to be a different kind of counsellor. Less rigid, more accessible. Warmer. More human.

That approach was critical to my work with Anna.

CHAPTER 7

Devon, July 2018

ANNA

As I left that first painful session, I resisted the overwhelming urge to sprint down the driveway towards the safety of my waiting family. I reached the car and caught sight of my reflection in the cobweb-covered wing mirror. Red-eyed and ashen-faced, I looked like I'd crawled out of the graveyard opposite. Wary of permanently scarring my children due to my appearance, I popped my sunglasses on and jumped in the car, immediately returning to 'mum mode'. I managed enthusiastic replies to my two-year-old's description of the gingerbread man he'd had at the local cafe and answered my six-year-old's questions about my 'appointment' – I told them I was seeing a physiotherapist for my shoulder.

'Does it hurt?' my seven-year-old asked.

More than you will ever know. 'No, Mummy's OK. Thank you, though.'

Only Sam knew where I had been and why. Knowing that it wasn't the time to ask how it had gone, he put a hand on mine, a small gesture which communicated everything he wanted to say in that moment: reassurance, empathy, warmth, kindness, compassion. Above all, safety. No words were needed.

Driving away, I could feel the anger building and swirling like a tornado inside me. I was furious for putting myself through that ordeal. I was overcome with embarrassment and intense shame. I knew I had shut down at the end of the session and just wanted to leave. I had told a complete stranger things that I'd spent half a life trying to hide. I deeply regretted opening my mouth and there was an overwhelming feeling that I was somehow in trouble. *He doesn't believe you. Stop being dramatic. What makes you so special to deserve any kindness?* My inner monologue was in full attack mode.

That night, even though I was physically and mentally exhausted, I couldn't sleep. Any sense of lightness I'd felt after finally being able to share my secret was overshadowed by humiliation and discomfort.

Desperate not to wake the children, I climbed wearily out of bed and stepped lightly across the landing, grabbing a couple of toddler-sized socks and almost tripping over a toy car on the way. Thinking that I might as well do something useful, I picked up the laundry basket, added the discarded clothes and crept down the stairs, taking care to avoid a creaky step. I loaded the washing machine, shoving as much as possible into the drum and sat down at the kitchen table. I watched the clothes circle around and around and combined with the gentle but continuous splashing, it became almost hypnotic. I sat there, wishing I could wash today's appointment away.

I replayed the session over and over in my head.

Although the therapist seemed really kind, I was worried. Did he think I was lying, like the others? Or if he believed me, did he think I was promiscuous and deserved it? Perhaps he thought it was a grey area? Why did he ask me about the police? Did he think that because I hadn't reported it, it didn't happen? Maybe he believed me but thought that I was evil for leaving a monster free to run around? My thoughts began to spiral.

The last few times I had told anyone what had happened, I would be so embarrassed I'd end up avoiding them – sometimes even ending friendships to protect myself from having to experience their reactions. Maybe it would be best not to return to counselling, so I wouldn't have to experience yet another bad reaction. I wasn't sure I could take it.

I didn't know whether Paddy even wanted me to make another appointment. Maybe I was incapable of being fixed and he could never help me. Perhaps no one could – I was too damaged, especially if I couldn't talk.

But I liked him, he seemed kind enough and I couldn't bear having to go through another first session with someone else. There were a lot of things I hadn't told this therapist yet. Even if he wanted me to return, was I brave enough to go back? I knew I still needed help.

I was worried about what Paddy thought of me. I wanted

him to understand that my behaviour that night had been so out of character. That I was a shy and studious person and I wouldn't normally have got that drunk or worn what I had. I was filled with shame, anger and self-hatred. I felt worthless. And although I was certain that if it had happened to someone else, I'd never blame them, I was consumed by guilt. Its shadowy blackness occupied every part of me, and I lived my life terrified and paranoid that my mortification was visible to everyone. I *knew* it was my fault and I felt annoyed when Paddy had repeatedly said it wasn't. I didn't understand how he could have read my words and believed I wasn't to blame.

He must have been irritated by my incessant fidgeting and lack of eye contact. I had tried to stop it, I really had. I hadn't meant to be defensive or resistant; I was just so petrified about confidentiality. I didn't want to get in trouble or be hurt. Could I trust him? I really wanted to and I desperately needed help. I just wasn't sure how to trust anyone other than Sam and a few close friends. I didn't even trust myself.

I was convinced Paddy thought I was rude and unappreciative and that he had more important things to do than deal with my many issues. I felt like such a burden to everyone. An inconvenience who was unworthy of help or kindness.

I hated the fact that what I'd told him was the only thing he knew about me. I was a normal, functioning, popular person, or so I thought. I didn't want to be 'brave'; I didn't want a 'well done for telling my story'. I didn't want a story – I wanted it to have never happened. If I didn't go back to therapy, I could carry on pretending I was 'fine'.

And the thing is, I had always been 'fine'. Until one day, I wasn't.

It was as though that first session had unlocked Pandora's box and although I tried to firmly shut it again, all the horrors of my past were straining and screaming against the lid, threatening to burst out.

I crept back up the stairs with the chirping of birds telling me that sunrise was imminent. I'd barely closed my eyes, when I heard the familiar sound of toddler footsteps running along the landing and charging in through the bedroom door. For a few blissful seconds, everything was normal. And then the painful hornet sting reminded me of the day before.

Overwhelmed by remorse and embarrassment, and absolutely horrified that I'd told a stranger about my private life, I emailed Paddy to say that I wouldn't be returning and I'd just pay him for the first session. I couldn't face him again.

———————————— " " ————————————

PADDY

At the end of the first session, it can be difficult to know what the client has made of the experience. Many things – politeness, nerves, a lack of confidence – can prevent them, particularly at this early point, from telling their counsellor how they really feel about the experience of therapy, especially if those feelings are negative. The days that follow the initial session, when thoughts, memories and emotions drift to a disrupted surface, can also shape their impressions. Inevitably, some elect not to return.

It was only the day after our session when I discovered what Anna was feeling. She emailed, telling me she was too ashamed and embarrassed to return. Usually, if a client stops therapy after just one appointment, I would respect their decision and autonomy, and beyond letting them know my door was open if they decided to return, I would not engage in further correspondence. Without the framework of a well-established therapeutic relationship, I have not earned the right to discuss their decision, what it might mean to them or whether it's the right one.

With Anna, it felt different. A part of her wanted to end the sessions, but another part of her wanted me to know how that first session had left her feeling. To me, it seemed like the beginning of a dialogue. I was also aware that she had taken an enormous step in coming to therapy and I didn't want that courageous act to be wasted and for her to abandon her journey at the first step. So, I replied swiftly. I told her that the feelings would pass and that by attending that first time, she had jumped a major hurdle, finding a way to talk about what had happened. I also reminded her that she had nothing whatsoever to feel ashamed about.

Later that day, Anna emailed again, confirming that she would return. She also paid for the second session in advance. It felt like she'd made a commitment.

For many counsellors, contact between sessions is usually only to arrange appointments, although some, like me, provide additional contact when necessary. While this is something that counsellor and client negotiate and agree on, with Anna, I made an intuitive, spur-of-the-moment decision. I felt that she needed reassurance and that her email required an immediate response.

Emails became a staple of our work together, a way to acknowledge the feelings and thoughts she had difficulty communicating in sessions. For a client who sometimes struggled to find her voice in person, Anna was a revelation in her messages. She was articulate and expressive, and I became convinced that if she could marry the person in those messages with how she presented in sessions, a powerful voice would emerge.

Anna was always at pains to stress that her emails did not require a response. Her respect for boundaries meant I was happy to respond. My instinct proved right. The exchanges were always brief. In essence, she needed to pin down her thoughts and feel the reassurance of an acknowledgement.

―――――――――――――― " " ――――――――――――――

ANNA

In his reply to my email, Paddy had kindly said that the embarrassment would pass, that I had nothing to feel ashamed of and that I had already done so well. It didn't feel like it, and I wasn't sure I believed him, but I appreciated his hopeful approach. I was surprised that he'd actually taken the time to reply and hadn't turned me away.

I was reminded once again of the myth of Pandora's box. After she couldn't contain her curiosity and opened it, Pandora unleashed evil into the world. But she became scared and quickly closed the box, trapping one spirit inside: hope.

Perhaps there was still hope for me. Maybe I could face the past. And perhaps I didn't have to do it alone.

CHAPTER 8

Bristol, July 2020

ANNA

Everything is familiar, but the events of that night seem so long ago that the city appears surreal. I can't believe we're actually here after planning it for so long and being confronted by so many obstacles.

Despite the map of Bristol seared into my brain, I pull up another one on my phone, just in case. Although it comforts me, I find that once we get going, I don't need it, as I remember a shortcut that leads us straight to my old university halls.

We're greeted by large, ugly metal gates, with vicious-looking spikes on top and a keypad to get in.

I'm immediately transported back to that night, running scared in the dark through the gates back to what was supposed to be a place of safety, yet being greeted by disbelieving and unsympathetic friends. I feel myself flood with shame as I recall the outfit I wore, despite it being a cold night. I become frustrated with myself for feeling ashamed and I force myself to focus.

Beyond the entrance, we see the unkempt campus, which doesn't appear to have moved on at all in twenty years. It's unclear whether the menacing gates are keeping something in or out.

I'm reminded of one of my four-year-old's favourite books *We're Going on a Bear Hunt* and the words, 'We can't go *over* it, we can't go *under* it, we'll have to go *through* it!' The thought of his giggles as I read to him makes me smile and brings me back to the present.

'Let's wait until someone comes out and we can nip in,' I suggest.

We stand hopefully at the gate, but no one comes. Just as I'm about to admit defeat and move on, I give the gates a solid push.

I look incredulously at Paddy as we realise the gates are unlocked and we walk straight through them and onto the campus.

Slowly and cautiously, I lead Paddy around the exterior of the halls until I reach the outside of my flat.

I stand motionless, staring at the normal-looking building. The word 'normal' keeps popping into my head. This place has haunted my dreams for the majority of my life. I've had flashbacks of the front door to my flat that evoked truly powerful and visceral fear. For months, I've worried about how I'd feel seeing this door again. And now I'm here, I don't feel anything.

Out of the corner of my eye, I can see Paddy looking at me, but I can't bear to return his gaze. I'm feeling something, but my brain is blocking it. Protecting me.

I don't know what you're supposed to feel when you visit a place of trauma with your therapist almost two decades later. The only thing I do know is that I'd trade anything to be someone else in this moment. To make everything disappear and to erase the past and my part in it.

CHAPTER 9

Greece, August 2018

PADDY

Shortly after Anna's first appointment, I went away with my family for a two-week holiday. The gap between sessions was not ideal. Anna had engaged, but I wondered whether, as the days slipped by, she might lose the courage to return.

The family trip was to a Greek island, a place we'd visited a number of times. In high season, it's full of families and over the years, the girls had made friends with other children. They often disappeared with their pals and we'd find them later in their favourite cafe, playing Uno and eating crêpes smothered with Nutella.

The island felt safe, a place where my wife and I could properly relax. It was the last place I ever expected to feel a sense of threat.

One morning, I was sitting on the hotel balcony. It was a

perfect time of day. A gentle breeze came in from the Aegean Sea and the sun was not yet fierce. Holidaymakers breakfasted in cafes along the waterfront and a ferry coming into harbour sounded its horn, the noise echoing around the bay.

I opened the BBC news app, intending to flick through the stories before heading to the beach to join my wife and daughters. Then, I saw the lead story.

The article was about Ampleforth, the previously all-male Catholic boarding school in north Yorkshire that I'd attended as a child. Once referred to as the Catholic Eton, Ampleforth's old boys include the Duke of Norfolk, Rupert Everett, David Stirling (the founder of the SAS), and King Letsie III of Lesotho. The piece revealed how the school had been singled out for investigation by the Independent Inquiry into Child Sexual Abuse (IICSA), set up in the wake of the Jimmy Savile scandal to identify where institutions had failed to protect the children in their care.

My first reaction was surprise. Beyond the casual acts of barbarity and predatory sexual behaviour that seem to be characteristic of all public schools, I hadn't noticed or experienced anything resembling abuse. As far as I knew, two monks at the school had been the subject of historic police investigations but given the emerging scale of abuse within the Catholic Church, those scandals seemed quite minor.

Yet, as I read the article, my surprise turned to horror. It spoke of physical and sexual abuse dating back to the 1960s that had affected boys as young as seven, of systemic issues that were known about at the highest levels of the school and beyond. I began to realise that it had been going on all around me – and would surely have affected students I'd known.

In an instant, I was back at Ampleforth, arriving for the very first time aged twelve. It was a damp autumnal afternoon. Towering Victorian architecture, all sharp gables and grimacing gargoyles. An abbey church as big and square and ugly as a power station. Long corridors of herringbone flooring that smelt of beeswax. Lugging a trunk up several flights of stairs to a dormitory with lofty ceilings and draughty windows. Cubicles with just a curtain for privacy. Older boys pointing and sneering and joshing together. A familiar voice inside – one I'd learned to ignore since I'd first started boarding at prep school aged seven – telling me that I was not safe.

Later, glimpsing the monks for the first time. Men in long black habits, who appeared to glide rather than walk.

On the hotel balcony, I downloaded the entire inquiry report and slowly read it all. By the time I reached the end, my shoulders were hunched and my neck was sore. I felt sick.

I spent the rest of the holiday thinking about what I'd read, wondering whether any of my friends had been abused. Wondering too what my elderly parents would have made of it but also finding ways to insulate myself against the revelations. They were too big and unwieldy. Instinctively, but certainly not consciously, I was trying to keep them at a safe distance.

When I returned from our holiday, I dropped in on my parents, who live close to me. I was a little startled to discover a copy of the *Telegraph* on their dining table, the paper open at a full-page spread about my school's abuse scandal.

'We kept this for you,' said my dad.

There was a neutrality to the comment and I wasn't quite sure what he was thinking.

I told them I'd read about it on holiday. 'It didn't happen to me,' I quickly added. 'It didn't happen to anyone I know.'

My parents were in their late eighties at the time. They'd read the *Telegraph*'s coverage, which was graphic enough. I couldn't see any point in confronting them with the scale of what I'd read in the report itself.

We discussed it for a short while. The atmosphere was subdued. It felt like we were sailing tentatively round the edges of an iceberg.

Mum and Dad are not stiff-upper-lipped types. There is love, warmth and humour in our relationship. But there's also a limit to the exchanges we have. They are products of their upbringing, class and generation. We do not talk about emotions.

Finally, I moved the conversation on, chatting about my holiday. The mood lifted.

Not long afterwards, I chanced on a clip of the LBC presenter James O'Brien on YouTube. He was a former pupil at the same school and he delivered a savage verdict on what had happened there.

'I feel such vicious anger at these men,' he said. 'Not only did they rape children and then cover it up; the people that never abused children are complicit in this in a way that I'm going to struggle to articulate. But every other parent that sent their child to this school has been robbed of pride in their own achievements. It makes me want to weep.'

Listening to him, a wave of emotion washed over me. He'd found words that I could not. It was an expression of pain, an emotion I was unable to access.

Why couldn't I feel anything as powerful?

Before long, the report's ghastly revelations receded to the back of my mind.

When my sessions with Anna began again shortly afterwards, I was more concerned with her search for resolution. Little did I know, she was bringing me closer to mine.

CHAPTER 10

'The act of revealing oneself fully to another and still being accepted may be the major vehicle of therapeutic help.'
IRVIN YALOM

PADDY

Although Anna had confirmed she would return for a second session, I was still relieved when I heard her knock on the door at the appointed time. It had been three weeks since we'd first met. Plenty of time for the shame and embarrassment she'd mentioned in her email to have overwhelmed her.

She looked pale and a little terrified as she sat across the room from me, perched on the edge of the sofa, as if ready to bolt.

I smiled, hoping my face communicated warmth and kindness and that Anna felt safe. 'How have you been?'

'OK,' she replied and handed me her phone again.

'Shall I read out loud?' I asked.

She shook her head vehemently.

I nodded back. I would keep her words to myself.

Anna had written about the shame again and how familiar an emotion it was. She described how confiding in friends about her experience always brought the same outcome: she was abruptly ghosted, as if she were a leper. Sometimes, she ended friendships herself, just so she could avoid the inevitable severance to come.

Anna believed that her story was toxic, that it drove people away. This seemed like a good moment to remind her that she was accepted and valued in the counselling space, no matter what she revealed. I looked up from her phone.

'This is a non-judgemental space, Anna,' I said. 'Nothing you say here will change that.'

———— " " ————

ANNA

I wouldn't have necessarily described myself as lacking in confidence or an anxious person. But my demeanour outside of the therapy room was a complete contrast to what Paddy witnessed for fifty minutes every week.

Before having children, I'd worked as a consultant in an engineering firm. I'd gained a master's degree, undertaking research and presenting my findings to academics and other influential people. I had many friends, was a good mum and was married to a loving man whom I'd been with since we were nineteen years old. But every time I sat on Paddy's couch, I was reduced to a shaking, mute mess. Unable to make eye contact or verbally communicate, I could barely look him in the eye, staring instead at his white Converse in an effort not to be truly seen.

My shame and embarrassment contributed to this, but there was also a deep-rooted fear of trust.

Letting Paddy in felt almost impossible. As the saying goes, 'trust is gained in drops and lost in buckets', and that had certainly been my experience with X.

The idea of relinquishing control felt absurd. I'd been hurt by someone I had deeply trusted. As a result, I'd put up a lot of sturdy and impenetrable barriers.

Of course, I had a 'professional' trust in Paddy. Logically, I knew he wouldn't hurt me, but while my head understood this, my heart and nervous system rarely agreed.

———————————— " " ————————————

PADDY

Given Anna's belief that her story had a destructive power, I felt it was necessary to remind her that it was safe with me, that it would not leak and poison the therapy space.

'As I've said before, these sessions are completely confidential. The only exceptions are when I speak with my supervisor, Sue, about my work – and she won't ever know your full name – or if I was concerned that you were in danger of hurting yourself or others.'

Tightly hunched over, Anna nodded silently in response. Like an animal that had just spotted a predator, she looked at me with wide, fearful eyes. Instead of reassuring her, I'd unwittingly thrown a grenade into the room.

———————— " " ————————

ANNA

In my head whirled a cacophony of thoughts and worries – a fear of opening up; a fear of being pushed away. Humiliation and discomfort tore through me like waves surging against a seawall. And then Paddy talked about confidentiality and my heart began to mimic the rhythm of my racing thoughts. What exactly did he mean by 'in danger of hurting yourself'?

The night before my second appointment, I was so utterly terrified and overwhelmed that I'd ended up self-harming.

As I got ready to leave for my session in the morning, I'd knocked over a cup of tea, the cold contents spilling over my skirt, and popped upstairs to change. Without thinking, I quickly dressed in front of Sam. I halted as I registered the shock, concern and horror on his face when he spotted the crop of fresh scratches on the top of my thigh. I burst into tears.

'I'm sorry,' I cried. I felt ashamed, disgusted and scared.

'It's OK,' he'd reassured me. 'Perhaps you could mention it to Paddy?'

An hour later, I again found myself squirming on Paddy's sofa. As he was discussing confidentiality, the words 'in danger of hurting yourself or others' echoed loudly in my head.

Of course, I'd previously trawled the internet to see if disclosing self-harm would get me into trouble, and the majority of posts I'd read suggested it was a very, very bad idea. I sat sobbing as I read stories of clients in the USA being committed to psychiatric hospitals and reported to the police. Then there were the horrific anecdotes of patients not offered pain relief while being stitched up in hospital.

I hadn't self-harmed since struggling to process my rapes at the age of eighteen, but in the months leading up to seeking therapy, I had relapsed twice. It had scared me and, ultimately, it was one of the catalysts for seeking help.

So, here I was sitting in front of a professional, torn between disclosing the information and the potential repercussions of doing so.

I waited until the session was nearly over before pulling out my phone again and placing it on the couch next to me. This was it, the thing that I most despised about myself. I had to take the risk that Paddy would either report me, section me or do something worse.

'I need to tell you something,' I fidgeted, vomit rising in my throat by the second. 'But I can't say it.'

'That's OK, take your time,' he said. The more anxious I became, the calmer he seemed to be. This didn't help – my jaw was clenched so tightly, the ball in my throat was so enormous that I was physically unable to speak. I was so terrified, I wanted to cry and run out of the room. *Remember why you're here. If you don't tell him, he can't help you.*

My breath had started to become jagged; my diaphragm was spasming.

'Just breathe,' he said.

I managed to calm my breathing down, but I'm not sure if it was due to pure willpower or the sheer embarrassment that I was being so dramatic in front of a stranger.

I decided it was now or never, reached for my phone and awkwardly stuck it out in front of me. As he leant forwards to take it, I hesitated.

'Are you sure?' he asked.

I could feel the tears welling up in my eyes as I handed him the phone. I held my breath. I was paralysed.

──────────────── " " ────────────────

PADDY

Slowly and hesitantly, Anna withdrew her arm, as if she was still debating whether to snatch the phone back. She looked at me, her eyes brimming with fear, like a child convinced they're in deep trouble. As it turned out, that assessment wasn't so far from the truth.

'Do you want me to read it out—' I stopped abruptly.

She was shaking her head tightly, her face barely moving an inch in either direction. It was a message communicated in the most minimal way, but the terror in those eyes told me everything I needed to know. That on no account was I to read the contents of her phone out loud.

There is something that I haven't told you – regarding why I have ended up seeking your help.

I told you that I'd had a flashback nightmare just before we met. I then woke up, threw up and had a panic attack on the bathroom floor. Then I said that I had cried myself to sleep.

However, after I'd been sick, I went downstairs and I ended up hurting myself. The next morning, I realised how pathetic it was, how much I detest it and that I don't want to do it ever again. It scares me.

I've also done this twice since I last saw you. I'm terrified that this means you will have to report me.

I feel like I'm eighteen again and experiencing everything for the first time, but now I'm in my thirties and I have responsibilities so I can't run away, get drunk or even be sad. This is the only thing that doesn't affect anyone else. I'm sorry I wasn't brave enough to tell you this.

" "

ANNA

As Paddy read, I searched his face for clues that I was in trouble. He handed me the phone back. Silence. *Say something!*

'OK,' he said. 'Thank you for telling me.'

What? What happens next?

'I'm really sorry. Sorry I couldn't tell you. Sorry, sorry... sorry,' I trailed off.

He held up his hands in an attempt to placate me.

'Do you have to report me?' I whimpered quietly, irritated at how pathetic I sounded.

'No, who would I report you to?' He almost looked amused. 'And you did tell me. Thank you.'

I let out a long exhale, relieved that I wasn't in trouble; I no longer had to carry the burden of this secret alone.

'It's OK,' he said. 'How did you hurt yourself?'

'Just my leg. It's only a scratch,' I replied, minimising it as much as possible. I knew this wasn't a coping mechanism that a seemingly responsible adult used.

Paddy ran through what sounded like a rehearsed list of dos and don'ts, but he managed to save it from being completely patronising by adding, 'But you're an educated and scientific woman. I know that you know all of this.' He seemed completely unfazed by what I'd told him and, most importantly, although I felt deeply ashamed, I didn't feel judged.

———————————— " " ————————————

PADDY

The debate surrounding self-harm is complicated and ever evolving. Ultimately, I can only ever respond to the person in front of me. If I sense they are in genuine danger, then of course I will act. I did not get that impression from Anna. For her, self-harm was a necessary mechanism. Complex, for sure, but only ever about coping.

It constituted such a small exchange at the end of a session in which we'd touched on so much more. But it was a significant one.

Self-harm remained one of Anna's greatest concerns, so I often returned to the same message of unfaltering acceptance. She repeatedly said that it was only when she finally managed to stop that she would be healed. As it turned out, her recovery took another form, making self-harm entirely redundant.

CHAPTER 11

ANNA

My introduction to self-harm was, perhaps, unusual. It wasn't something that I had discovered myself, seen on TV, read about or had ever considered. It was, however, another instance of pain at the hands of a man. Let's call him J.

It was 2002 and I was sitting on a rotting wooden bench outside a nightclub in Devon. A few days before, I had been alone in my university flat in Bristol, packing to go home for the summer. The doorbell rang and, without checking the peephole, I opened the door. X forced his way into my home and raped me again.

The nightclub's gutters rattled to the drum and bass booming from within. The vibrations made the bench and my head pound. I looked down at the zebra-print bottle, containing some sort of alcopop, in my hand. I wondered how I'd ended up here. It seemed so long ago that I'd left home and headed to Bristol for the first time. Barely eighteen years old, I was full of hope and excitement for a new life. Now I was sad and bitter that the academic year had ended like this.

That evening, I'd met up with friends hoping to drink the pain away but quickly realised that being drunk wouldn't solve anything. In fact, I needed to stay in control.

My friends were keen to share stories from their first year at various universities around the UK. The drunken adventures, the relationships that had been formed – or dissolved – all the mistakes they'd made and learned from along the way. The normality of life. It had been the worst year of mine, but I joined in and pretended otherwise.

Anticipating comments about my physical appearance – gaunt and pale, make-up hiding the colourful bruises that swirled beneath my skin – I blamed my state on partying too hard at the summer ball, thus safely masking my suffering.

Most of us had left the apparent safety of student halls and were moving into houses at the end of the summer. My friends thought they were grown up. I didn't know whether I was, or wanted to be, grown up or not. I wasn't sure I had a choice.

The only thing I knew was that I had to keep my mouth shut. I couldn't tell anyone what had happened and I hoped that if I didn't think about it, it would just go away.

Suddenly, the drum and bass became louder as someone opened the door and lurched heavy-footed down the steps.

Even though I hadn't seen or spoken to J in at least six

months, his familiarly offensive aftershave announced his arrival. He sat down clumsily next to me, resting his head on my shoulder.

'I still think about you,' he slurred.

I shuddered and shifted along the bench, away from him. J and I had briefly dated and he was one of the few people I'd spoken to about the first rape. At the time, his reaction had been cold and cruel. Although I was now determined to keep my mouth shut, perhaps on some self-destructive level I was seeking a similar response. Out it tumbled. 'It happened again,' I said without emotion, staring straight ahead.

He leant forwards, burying his head in his hands. I wasn't sure if he was attempting to be sympathetic or was about to puke. I didn't care either way.

'Jesus,' he eventually managed to reply. He gave the bare minimum, as always.

Neither of us spoke as there was a lull in the music and the reverberating gutter was quiet for a moment, providing my head with some welcome relief, before the next track began and the crowd loudly cheered. I began to tremble and shake in time with the music.

'I have something that'll help fix you,' he said, putting an arm around my shoulders.

Assuming he meant either sex or drugs, I started to protest. I wasn't interested. Not in drugs and definitely not in him.

'Your loss,' he shrugged, draining the last of the beer from the dirty brown glass bottle he was holding. It looked ugly compared to the black-and-white zebra stripes of my bottle, and even uglier because he was holding it. I thought I was indifferent towards J, but at that moment, I *hated* him. Suddenly, he smashed the bottle against the side of the bench and glanced around to see if anyone had seen. Confident that no one was around, he picked up a piece of glass, grabbed my tiny wrist and sliced into my bare arm before I could process what was happening. I froze in disbelief and stared down at the deep incision, about two inches long, on my forearm. The blood quickly trickled down to my wrist, soaked my friendship bracelet and began to blanket the palm of my hand.

I felt nothing. There was no physical pain, at least initially, as I detached from my body. It was as though I was looking at someone else's arm, like I was watching the interaction through a television screen.

He handed me another piece of glass and I saw myself reach out and take it, feeling like I was fully on autopilot. He gestured for me to cut. And I did. Without caring, without thinking of the consequences, I did. I didn't want to, but I didn't know what else to do.

CHAPTER 12

'It is the client who knows what hurts, what directions to go, what problems are crucial, what experiences have been deeply buried. It began to occur to me that unless I had a need to demonstrate my own cleverness and learning, I would do better to rely upon the client for the direction of movement in the process.'

CARL ROGERS

PADDY

Anna had experienced the very worst of humanity and was understandably extremely wary of letting me in. So, how was I going to win her trust?

In those initial sessions, my instinct was that she did not need fancy therapeutic interventions. She simply needed to feel that she was in a safe place, with a man she could trust.

During those sessions, when Anna continued to communicate via her phone, I went back to the very basics of my training, to the core conditions of empathy and unconditional positive regard.

Empathy appears to be all the rage these days. It's gone from a social media buzzword to a corporate leadership tool. That's ultimately a positive development, but I wonder if its meaning has been slightly misinterpreted or even lost in the process.

To me, empathy is the ability to understand a person's feelings and experience from their unique point of view.

Empathy is not sympathy, although the two are closely related.

Sympathy often contains a trace of pity. Picture two friends – Tom and Jane – in conversation. 'I've split up with Ed,' says Tom tearfully. 'You poor thing,' replies Jane. 'You must be heartbroken.' It's not the worst response, but in addition to her pity, she's made an assumption; Tom has yet to tell her exactly where his sadness lies. Sympathy can also have an element of personal experience. So, Jane might choose to tell Tom about a break-up she's been through: 'I know just how you feel. I was inconsolable for months.' There may even be a whiff of judgement – 'You should have left him years ago' – as well as advice: 'What you need is a night out, to put all this behind you.'

If she was reacting empathetically, Jane would respond by meeting her friend where he is. 'I'm so sorry, Tom. You seem very upset.' She'd make him feel heard and in doing so, invite him to reveal more of what he's experiencing and what, in particular, his tears are expressing, which might be sorrow but equally might also be rage or relief. In time, he'd feel seen (because Jane has acknowledged the unique place in which he finds himself) as well as a powerful sense of connection. His friend Jane has taken the time to truly understand.

Carl Rogers, the American psychologist who pioneered the person-centred therapeutic approach in the 1940s, believed empathy to be the most important aspect of counselling: 'To my mind, empathy is in itself a healing agent. It is one of the most potent aspects of therapy, because it releases, it confirms, it brings even the most frightened client into the human race. If a person is understood, he or she belongs.'

In my relationship with Anna, empathy was about communicating that I understood her world through my words, responding in ways that showed her I had actively listened. It was also about my body language.

So, when Anna sat hunched on the edge of the sofa, I maintained an open posture, my arms uncrossed. I nodded when she spoke, my face communicating the emotion of my response along with my words. Eye contact was important too, but with Anna, who often preferred to stare at my shoes, I adopted a measured approach, so she didn't feel overly scrutinised.

In those early weeks, Anna turned up for sessions wracked with shame about the content she'd shared the previous week. It was imperative she understood that my acceptance of her and her experience would not change, whatever she brought me, however she behaved. To this end, I offered what Rogers refers to as unconditional positive regard – treating her with the same warmth and kindness each week, so she knew that what she'd told me was heard without judgement.

There was also the need to communicate that I accepted the truth of her account, particularly when new facets were introduced. And so, whenever appropriate, I repeated three words, which I hoped might one day sink in: 'I believe you.'

While Anna slowly became more comfortable in the sessions, fidgeting less and making some eye contact, the state of deep trust in which she felt entirely secure and safe in the therapeutic relationship – and truly believed that I believed her – took months, if not years, to achieve.

I distinctly remember an early session when the process of building that all-important bond was very nearly derailed.

―――――――――――― " " ――――――――――――

ANNA

The therapy process felt very precarious to me, like Jenga; one bad session, one instance of sharing too much, and the entire structure would topple.

Paddy saw a supervisor every month and discussed his work with her. I knew that, like my sessions with him, those discussions were confidential. Yet for me, there was a substantial difference between knowing that he was going to see her and finding out that he actually had.

'I spoke with Sue, my supervisor, about our work,' he said at the start of one session, when it was obvious that, once again, I was struggling to find the words.

'So, she knows what happened to me?'

'She does. She supported many women who've been through similar experiences when she worked for Women's Aid.'

I think he meant to be reassuring. But I didn't feel reassured. I began to squirm on the sofa. *Fuck. I bet she's judged me, reminded him that 'some women cry rape', pointed out the holes in my story because I can't remember important details like dates or what trousers X was wearing.*

'OK, did she say anything helpful? Is there a plan moving forward?' I asked, attempting to be positive. *What the fuck did he tell her? I don't know this woman and I didn't decide to tell her the graphic details of my life. What has Women's Aid got to do with anything? I'm not a victim. Keep calm, professional. Get through this session.*

'There isn't really a plan... erm, I guess we just stumble forwards?'

He said it uncertainly, shifting a little in his armchair, his hand reaching up to rub his neck.

I handed over my phone. For the rest of the session, he read the notes I'd written and offered some observations, but there was a disconnect. I didn't know what I was feeling until later that day and I realised that, for the first time, I was angry. Angry at Paddy, angry at his supervisor, angry at myself. I'd left the session with a curt and uncharacteristic, 'Thanks. Goodbye.' Yet politeness and people-pleasing were deeply rooted in the core of my being and I was utterly embarrassed at the manner in which I'd ended the session.

That night, Sam and I had put the kids to bed and headed downstairs to crash on the sofa in front of another episode of *Black Mirror*, both of us exhausted from the day. Toys were scattered on the floor and the dinner dishes still needed to be done, yet I'd found myself sitting down.

'How did it go today?' Sam asked, plonking himself down next to me on the sofa before quickly adding, 'You don't have to tell me, just know that I'm here if you want to talk.'

I let out a long sigh and crinkled my nose, burying my head in my hands.

'I was really rude to Paddy today.'

'I'm sure you weren't,' he said, turning to face me.

'I was,' I said, refusing to return his stare. 'I didn't want to talk to him and I left without really saying goodbye. It's like I was a moody teenager.' *This was quite the understatement; I even ignored Lola on the way out.*

Sam moved closer and pulled me into a hug. I stared straight ahead at a framed photo of the Grand Canyon. Happy memories of a three-week trip we'd taken across the USA in our mid-twenties. Before therapy and the endless curse of self-analysis.

'Do you think that maybe because you'd made really good progress last week, you somehow don't deserve to have positive feelings? And now you're on your own self-sabotage mission, wanting to push the people who are trying to help you away?'

'Maybe,' I offered, moving away from his arms and

inadvertently proving his point. *Definitely. When did he become a therapist?*

I stood up and assessed the mess on the floor. 'I wrote some stuff down about how I was angry that he'd spoken to his supervisor and that I'm really pissed off that we have to "stumble forwards" with no plan. I know it's completely illogical.'

'I'll sort the toys later. Did you tell him?'

I bent down, noticing a twinge in my back – the result of years of rocking babies and toddlers to sleep in my arms – and started to pick up a few puzzle pieces and arrange them back together.

'No, I couldn't make sense of my emotions when I was with him. All I knew was that I wanted to leave. I thought I'd be happy having two therapists working to support me, but I actually feel betrayed, judged and angry.'

Sam bent down to help and for a few minutes we silently tidied away the day's chaos.

'Maybe you could just tell him that and send him the angry note to explain what was going on for you?' he said, carefully lining up some toy cars on the shelf. 'It might help.'

I returned Peppa Pig to her rightful place – a shoebox bed that I'd made with my youngest that day.

'He'll probably say it's projection and I'm angry at the wrong people,' I said, covering Peppa with a tiny blanket.

'And if he said that, would he have a point?'

'Maybe.' *Definitely.*

I found the last piece under the sofa and as I completed

the puzzle of Pedro Pony and his friends, I began to wonder whether I'd ever be able to piece myself back together. Perhaps there would always be pieces missing, or perhaps the pieces were now too misshapen, ruined by the past and no longer able to fit together.

--- " " ---

PADDY

Keeping Anna engaged in her therapy was of paramount importance. But my mention of Sue had rattled her, as had my comment about stumbling forwards. It felt like another mistake. She was paying to see me every week and was fully entitled to expect a structure to future sessions, but I'd given her the impression that I planned to just feel blindly for the path ahead. I also wondered whether my wishy-washy answer had horrified her engineer's brain, which was more comfortable in the precise, quantifiable world of mathematics and physics.

I'd watched as she retreated further into herself during the session, her face pinched, her voice tight. The following day, an email arrived from her, in which she apologised for being rude and explained why. She included a screenshot of a note she'd written, in which she conveyed her feelings about the session more honestly. It was an interesting contrast. A polite email and the more direct, uncensored language of her note. It was as if she wanted to express anger but good manners held her back. In time, I hoped she'd be able to find that pure expression in the sessions. But for now, I had enough information to know what had happened.

I typed a reply, even though she'd not asked for one.

Hi Anna,

I'm so sorry you felt this way yesterday. I sensed things weren't right, so thank you for letting me know why.

I can well imagine how you might have felt when I told you about my supervisor. It's another person knowing, when you've spent so long keeping your experience in the most private of places. All I can say is that my supervisor is a calm, kind, wise therapist with years and years of experience. She understands – completely – the importance of confidentiality. She is without judgement and, as I said, has worked for Women's Aid, which means she has spoken to many women who have had experiences similar to yours. It's really important I discuss my work with her because I want to make sure I am helping you in the best way possible. I wanted to be transparent with you, but I can understand how that might have been scary.

Getting annoyed with your counsellor is quite normal. It's actually healthy. No need to apologise. My Jungian psychoanalyst used to annoy the crap out of me! We can discuss all those points next time. 'Stumbling forwards' was a clumsy phrase. But yes, there is not a rigid plan. I need to meet you where you are each week, which demands a degree of flexibility. I hope that makes sense.

All I can do is repeat what I always say (boring and repetitive, I know): You are doing phenomenally well. You have started to face the most difficult events of your life. It is so hard for you. There's a reason you kept them sealed in a bunker in your head for seventeen years. There are bound to be moments when the pain of looking at them is unbearable; when you glimpse happiness but perhaps – I'm guessing now – don't feel that you deserve it and decide to self-sabotage. And I totally understand why you would want to push your therapist away. Just so you know, I am not going anywhere. So, if you can face it, I will see you on Tuesday at 5 p.m.

Paddy

It was one of many ruptures and repairs along the way, moments where the relationship was briefly damaged and where effort was made on both sides to heal. I was more than happy to write those emails, to do whatever it took to bring Anna back to counselling. To show her that she could reveal herself in therapy and, unlike her friends, I would not turn my back.

CHAPTER 13

Bristol, July 2020

ANNA

As we stand outside the flat, looking at its weathered exterior, a train thunders past nearby, making my heart pound and the hairs on the back of my neck stand up. I briefly get drawn into a flashback of hearing a train *that* night.

And, as if cruelly scripted, I feel it. Starting in my torso, it spreads under my ribcage like a poisonous creeping vine, sucking away my breath and any remaining confidence. It unfurls inside my throat, forcing it to constrict and stealing my voice. I can feel it behind my eyes and in the dilated blood vessels of my reddening cheeks. It moves insidiously down my lower body into the ground, rooting me to the spot.

Unstoppable shame.

I'm ashamed of what happened to me and I'm embarrassed that Paddy knows the graphic details of what occurred inside the walls of the drab brick building we're staring at. Most of all, I'm ashamed of being me.

I'm trying not to get pulled into and lost among the memories, and I'm comforted by Paddy being nearby. I remind myself that I'm safe and that I can do this. I haven't come this far to only come this far.

We've travelled almost a hundred miles to visit this place. I've spent two long and painful years in therapy and we've planned this trip in granular detail. We've spent months talking about the 'what ifs'. I know I can do this. The shame may feel unstoppable, but so am I.

I'm full of hope that this trip will have a positive outcome. Will I finally be able to put these events in the past? Will I be able to get some resolution and closure? To move on and reclaim my life? I want this more than anything and I know my therapist feels the same.

———————————— " " ————————————

PADDY

We've had many long discussions about this trip, covering Anna's fears, expectations and hopes for the day, as well as what she'd like me to bring to the process. We have done everything we can to ensure we take our therapeutic bubble with us on this journey, so as we walk the streets of Bristol, we remain in the safe space that we've nurtured together over the previous two years.

I managed to contain my fears in the car, but as we arrived in the city, passing through suburbs and into the centre, they hit with force. My pulse began to race and my hands, now clammy, clutched the steering wheel too tightly. In that moment, it struck me how ridiculously ambitious, to the point of foolhardy, it was to assume that we could replicate our bubble in the middle of Bristol. This is a city with a large population and we were entering the very heart of it. How were we supposed to maintain our safe space navigating Bristol's public areas? There were interactions to come. Encounters we could avoid; others, inevitably, that we could not. All of this required energy and micro-decision-making.

I went back to basics, quietly taking a series of slow, deep breaths. Gradually, I began to calm down. The preparation included contingencies for almost every possible outcome. And besides, Anna and I weren't strangers. After two years, we communicated with each other effectively. If something truly unexpected occurred, we'd find a way to work through it.

By the time we're standing outside Anna's flat, my fears have abated. Like us, the city has only just emerged out of lockdown and it appears that most of its inhabitants have decided to stay at home. Our bubble, for now at least, is secure.

I can concentrate on Anna, which is just as well. As I glance in her direction, I notice a slight tightness has settled over her face, a pinching around the eyes. Her skin has drained of colour.

Is she dissociating? Within the context of my counselling room, with her seated directly in front of me, the signs are easy to spot. But we're not in the counselling room any more. Now, she's standing beside me in profile, in an urban environment full of distractions, not least the trains that regularly pass behind us. I don't want to disturb her if I'm wrong, but if I'm right, I need to find a way to convince her that she's safe to return to the present.

I'm anxious again. Is this all too much for Anna? Is the weight of being here – the landscape of her nightmares experienced in the cold, unforgiving light of day – about to crash down on us both?

" "

ANNA

I need to move. To *do something*. I take a couple of tentative steps towards the building before retreating back to the safety of my therapist. Small steps.

The building bears the scars of neglect, its surface marred by peeling paint and graffiti tags. Battle wounds.

Now, Paddy is looking directly at me and I still can't bear to connect. If he says something empathic or tells me it wasn't my fault (because he likes to repeat himself), I'll either break down and cry or punch the wall in front of me. Luckily, he says nothing and the swirling mess of emotions passes while I stare at the depressing grey-brick wall directly ahead to distract myself. I pull at the weeds growing out of the cracks and notice that a solitary dandelion has managed to flower. It seems so obviously out of place and symbolic that I'm annoyed at the metaphor that pops into my head: how even in the darkest of places, hope can grow. The clichédness of it all pisses me off and I rip the flower out of the brickwork. I immediately feel guilty. Sad. Stupid. I've always struggled to express my anger and now I feel utterly guilty and ridiculous taking it out on a flowering weed.

I hope Paddy doesn't know what I'm thinking. This is unlikely, as usually he knows me better than I do. Just in case, I deflect onto another topic and start rambling about the time my friend got drunk, became overconfident about her rollerblading skills and tumbled dramatically down the steps we're standing by, while somehow remaining unscathed. I'm not sure what the point of my story is, but I'm trying to lighten the mood. I don't succeed. On the surface, I'm presenting with all the confidence of my drunken rollerblading friend, but actually I'm not as indestructible as I pretend to be, and as Paddy gives me a confused look, I know I'm not convincing him.

———————————— " " ————————————

PADDY

I'm grateful Anna has said something. Her delivery is speedy, her anxiety pressing a foot to the pedal, but she appears to be on the ground, not floating above where we stand. She's telling a story about then. She's able to be here.

———————— " " ————————

ANNA

Up until this moment, defiance and courage have helped me focus on the flats. But now, every instinct is telling me to avert my gaze, as if the very act of looking will unravel my composure. Following a primal urge to shield myself from pain, my eyes dart round trying to find something else to lock on to. I'm reminded of Carl Jung's quote: 'That which you most need will be found where you least want to look.' I want to tell Jung, respectfully, to piss off. I'm trying.

I take in my surroundings. I'd forgotten how frequent and loud the trains were. There are no other students here and everything seems dead and deserted, as if for our benefit. I spot some opportunistic seagulls fighting near a discarded bin bag and their screeches remind me of being at home, near the sea in Devon. It's strangely comforting. I look down at my feet and as I kick the loose gravel, I'm reminded of the first six months of my therapy, in which I could only manage to look at Paddy's white Converse.

I realise that I've been silent for a few minutes. After two years of sessions, I'm pretty good at holding silences, but I really want to get the most out of being here. I take a gamble and articulate my thoughts.

'I feel conflicted. I want to both look and not look at the flats,' I tell him. I'm struggling to communicate what I mean and my delivery is clumsy, but it has broken the silence.

'But you have been staring at the building since we arrived,' he points out.

It's not quite what I meant, but I go along with it and feel a glimmer of pride as I realise he's right. I think about how far I've come. I wouldn't have been able to make this trip a year ago or at any time over the past two decades. Maybe Jung had a point.

I realise that this is the first time I've been back here since those events. I'd been to other parts of the city in the past few years, which had certainly been triggering, but I'd never returned here. I'm strangely calm and I sense that there is a separation between now and then. I begin to feel in control, which surprises me. Alongside this there is sadness and I'm not sure if it's for the eighteen-year-old I was or for the life I should have had.

" "

PADDY

She's been silent for several minutes, her arms tightly crossed as though trying to keep something in or something out. I'm confident she's not dissociating, but I wonder whether she needs a gentle reminder that she's not alone.

" "

ANNA

'What's going on for you right now?' Paddy asks.

'I feel... responsible.' My flat door, which once represented endless possibilities when I crossed it as a fresher, now seems like a barrier separating me from happiness. I'd left at the end of my first year through the same door, scarred and changed for ever.

'I opened the door and let him in. I didn't check the peephole.' A sliding-doors moment. The worst mistake of my life.

'It was a split-second decision,' he says. 'The kind people make every day. How could you possibly have known what was to come?'

I open my mouth to argue but stop myself. He has a point. Perhaps there wasn't much I could have done to prevent X. Of course, this isn't the first time we've had this discussion, but for some reason standing here now, I fully hear it. I don't need Paddy to verbalise it, I know what he's saying: *I'm not to blame.* I repeat it over and over in my head. *I'm not to blame. It wasn't my fault.* I ignore any thoughts that try to convince me otherwise.

I think I'm ready to leave. I look at the flats one last time and draw in a deep breath, raising my shoulders and expanding my chest. I count to ten and exhale. The breath leaves my lips forcefully, carrying with it accumulated memories and turbulent narratives.

And while I may be changed for ever by what transpired within those walls, I imagine a different ending to my story.

I walk out of the door, leaving the terror behind. I remember the tenacity of the dandelion pushing its way through the cracked wall and feel a flicker of resilience ignite and build with each imaginary step away. I have a new-found strength and compassion for myself.

'Shall we move on?' I suggest.

'If you're ready?'

I give a firm nod.

CHAPTER 14

'Dreams are the facts from which we must proceed.'
CARL JUNG

ANNA

'How has your week been?'

Sessions often began along this line of enquiry. A seemingly straightforward question, yet that day it made my stomach violently churn and release a kaleidoscope of butterflies. I swallowed to prevent myself from vomiting and looked towards the map on the wall.

The week had been brimming with vivid and violent nightmares and I was haunted by images that seemed to erupt from the infernos of hell. When I woke, terrified and confused, these visions faded, yet they would leave me with lingering feelings of unease and disgust. I couldn't make sense of them. Nonetheless, I was pleased to have had a dream that I remembered in its entirety and wasn't too embarrassed to share.

Pulling my sleeves down over my hands, I stared at the map on the wall. *Be brave. Say something.*

'I had a dream last night and wrote it down.'

Paddy suddenly became animated and reached for a pen and paper. 'You mind if I make notes?'

---- " " ----

PADDY

I first became interested in dreams and their power to illuminate therapeutic work when I was seeing Philip, the Jungian psychoanalyst, in my twenties. I remember the very first dream I took to him, which featured an amalgam of my childhood homes.

My father was an army officer and I was mostly brought up on military bases, where I lived during the holidays when I wasn't away at boarding school. I remember those army quarters as bland, regimented properties, which my mother kept very tidy. The gardens were similarly neat, stripped of abundance, colour and life and were ideal for tenants who never stayed long enough to invest in planting.

In my dream, while the house remained orderly, the garden was wild and overgrown, a snagging tangle of brambles and out-of-control weeds.

Philip helped me to look at my dreams through Jung's analytical lens. It remains for me one of the most powerful pieces of therapeutic learning.

Jung believed that dreams are spaces in which the unconscious draws on the imagery of the everyday to symbolise emotions or desires. So, while dreams can appear to be filled with fantastical or illogical vignettes and scenes, they are, in fact, rich in content and meaning.

Jungian dream analysis begins by considering every element – the setting, people, objects, smells, tastes, colours, light, dialogue, quite literally everything that can be recalled – in the hope that associations (such as memories, thoughts and sensations) can be made. Importantly, in dreams, real people do not represent their real-life counterparts. So if, for example, you dream about a selfish friend, it's likely that you're dreaming about a selfish part of you. Once you have established your associations, an interpretation can sometimes emerge. It's one that will likely feel revelatory and shed light inwards.

With Philip's help, I saw that my dream about the tangled garden was about two contrasting worlds. The house – with its neat, subdued interior – represented a way of thinking I'd inherited from my childhood. There was plenty of love as I grew up, but there was also a sense of emotions being kept in check. When I began boarding at the age of seven, I learned to shut down my feelings, a process compounded by life at my prep school, where the Jesuits enthusiastically dished out beatings for the most minor misdemeanours and Catholicism – with its emphasis on sin and repression – permeated the very air. The garden, by contrast, represented freedom. The brambles and weeds were a sign of emotional abundance and, for want of a better word, mess.

There was something profoundly comforting about this interpretation. It was OK to feel.

———————————— " " ————————————

ANNA

'We were in a garden together somewhere,' I began. 'You and I. There was pink blossom hanging between us, obstructing my view of you.'

I suddenly felt a little foolish hearing my words aloud.

'Pink blossom,' he repeated quietly to himself as he wrote.

'You handed me a giant chalkboard and although you didn't say anything or give instructions, I somehow knew that I was supposed to write a list of all the good and bad things about myself. I drew a line down the middle of the board, so that the left column took up the majority of the space. I started by listing the "good" things, and on the right-hand side of the chalkboard, I wrote: "caring, loving, trustworthy and a good friend". And then I crossed out "a good friend". I knew the other column would be much longer and luckily, I woke up before I had to write it.'

Paddy carefully set the biro down and studied his words, tilting his head slightly. He held the page away from him, at arm's length, as if seeking an additional perspective. This was a new dynamic between us – usually he waited for me to say something and now, I was eager to hear his thoughts.

'Can I offer some observations?'

'Please.' *Anything is better than silence.*

'OK, although there's a barrier between us, it's delicate. It could easily be brushed aside. It's not a stone wall.'

'Hmm.' *He means I'm starting to let him in.* I wasn't sure whether I was happy with this, but it seemed to be happening regardless.

'Secondly, you've chosen to write in chalk, which is something that can be easily rubbed out and changed.'

'That's true.' *It seemed obvious now that he'd said it.*

'But even though you could have rubbed out "good friend", you chose to cross it out, leaving it visible, perhaps suggesting that a part of you still believes you are a good friend?'

He made it sound very simple and neat, which was the complete opposite to the way my brain usually supplied my thoughts. Perhaps my unconscious wasn't as stupid as I thought.

'It's only one interpretation,' he offered. 'If you feel it fits, then perhaps it's helpful.'

My analysis had been that I had too many bad qualities to fit on a chalkboard and I was thankful I'd woken up before I had to write them down. But throughout the day, my conscious brain had then provided me with a long list nonetheless. So I was grateful for Paddy's fresh perspective.

Dreams became a useful way to communicate my fears and make the unconscious conscious, allowing us to explore it.

* * *

I remember another session around six months into my work with Paddy. I'd started to open up and was less reliant on the notes on my phone to speak to him. I had even begun to piece together the events of twenty years ago and compile an account of them.

It was a freezing cold February morning and as I cautiously made my way up the icy drive, I couldn't help but compare this day to that of my first appointment. Although my nerves still jangled as I walked up the path to every session, I had begun to feel some sense of progress. And whereas on that first day I trudged up the drive with my head down, almost afraid to take up space in the world, I was now able to spot signs of beauty and appreciate them. The sunlight caught the frost that sparkled on the branches like nature's glitter and I instinctively pulled out my phone to take a photograph. Capturing this beauty through my lens calmed me and arrested the thoughts that I had replayed on the journey here. I'd woken early that morning, terrified and confused by a dream that I couldn't seem to stop thinking about.

I'd barely sat down on the couch in my usual spot – the furthest away from Paddy's chair – before I launched into recollecting the dream. As I started to speak, he quickly reached for something to write with.

'I was on a train with lots of carriages. You were at one end; my family was at the other. I ran down the train, but by the time I'd got to them, their carriage had been removed and so I ran back down to yours, which by then had also been removed. The carriages kept disappearing one by one, until there were only two left – the one I was standing in, and a horrible dark carriage that I'd managed to avoid by climbing over every time I ran up and down the train. I didn't want to go into the dark one in case the carriage I was in disappeared and I was stuck there. Alone.'

Paddy set down his pen. 'Can I offer some thoughts?'

'Sure, although I think I've figured some of it out. The dark carriage represents my trauma and I spent the whole dream trying to avoid it and running between you, or therapy, and my family.'

He nodded. 'Makes sense. I also wonder whether there is still some shame for you about being in therapy and you want to keep those two aspects of your life separate from each other?'

'Definitely. The carriage is in the middle, so I guess I'm trying to keep both my family and you away from it.'

At this point, I had yet to tell Paddy the details of what had happened to me and I was terrified to do so. How could I learn to trust again when I had obviously shown such poor judgement of people in the past?

'Rest assured, Anna, that when you step into that dark carriage, you don't have to do it alone. I'll be by your side.'

CHAPTER 15

PADDY

Understanding my dream about the bramble-filled garden had freed me in psychoanalysis. No longer inhibited by the repressed thinking I'd inherited from my childhood, I felt able to explore my time at boarding school. But the more I looked at the period I'd spent away from home, the less comfortably it sat with me.

I began boarding aged seven and finished when I was seventeen. Ten years, of which I spent the majority away from my family.

I remember leaving therapy one evening. It was autumn and while I'd been inside with Philip, the day outside had begun to draw to a close. The streetlights on Haverstock Hill were blinking into life as a chill wind sent leaves skittering along the pavement.

I was about to walk down the hill to Belsize Park Tube Station when I spotted a mum with her young son strolling towards me. The boy, who wore a school uniform and was aged around seven or eight, was clinging to her hand and chatting away.

I felt a sudden jolt of discomfort, like I'd touched an electric fence. I stood stock-still as they walked past.

It was as if someone had held up a mirror, showing me the boy I was when I was sent away.

I pictured him being left at a strange new school, his beloved mother driving off. It was heartbreaking to contemplate.

'Too young,' I muttered to myself, the words catching in my throat. 'Too young.'

It was the first time I'd connected to the child I was then. The first time I'd seen him clearly. Seen how little he was and how devoted he was to his mother. She was his everything.

As the months slipped by in that airless therapy room in Hampstead, what had previously been fuzzy and out of reach was brought into sharp definition. Where before I could only picture the superficial details of my life back then – the blazer and tie I wore, the arcane, illogical rules to which I had to adhere, the faces of teachers and peers – other memories, once buried deep, now rose to the surface.

The first day. A mix of bewilderment and devastation as I said goodbye to my parents in the formal entrance hall of my prep school, an austere red-brick Victorian building near Windsor.

I'd never been away from home before. Never been separated from my parents. One minute they were there, giving me a kiss, the next they were gone. I had known this moment was coming for weeks and had anticipated it with a jumble of nerves and dread, but the reality was a very different beast.

My older brother was there to help me settle in. We carried my trunk upstairs to the dormitory and he showed me where the showers and toilets were. Although his presence was supportive and comforting, it was also disconcerting. The fact that he was still boarding, three years after he entered the school, suggested to me that this was an irreversible decision. I was stuck there and that moment of clarity crystallised into a feeling of profound abandonment.

The sensation lingered for weeks. Possibly longer. But it paled in comparison to the desolation I experienced, an emotion that twisted my stomach and made my seven-year-old heart hurt. Those who've been educated in the boarding school system typically call it 'homesickness', but when I think of the deep sadness that engulfed me after the lights were turned out, it seems a rather tame word.

The dormitory was about fifty metres long, lined on both sides with dozens of cubicles which had curtains that could be drawn across the front, the only privacy we were afforded. I learned to cry quietly – already aware that I had to keep my despair to myself if I was to survive this experience – although other boys were less restrained. I remember one pupil from Saudi Arabia who wept loudly into the night, prompting jeers and name-calling. He was also a regular bed-wetter who had to suffer the indignity of having his sheets stripped in the morning by a tutting matron.

I had brought a teddy from home. Fozzie Bear, a character from the Muppets, had a little plastic pork-pie hat, a polka dot necktie and a permanent grin. I needed him to be happy, because I was anything but. In the middle of the night, I used to whisper in his ear, asking him to relay messages to my other teddies at home. I was, I see now, desperate to connect to the world I'd been torn from.

I recently unearthed the letters I sent home at that time. My handwriting is joined up and immaculate and in one I proudly declare that I'm not homesick any more. I was already learning to shut down emotionally, to accept my new life, even if, at some unfathomably deep level, I was still in pain.

The people now responsible for my care were the Jesuits, a religious order founded by St Ignatius of Loyola in 1540. They wore black suits and shirts, with a square of white at the collar to indicate their priestly status. When I've spoken to friends educated by Catholic orders, the Christian Brothers emerge as the most violent and sadistic of them by far. But the Jesuits also knew a thing or two about inflicting pain. These men of God were infamous for designing their very own version of a cane. The ferula was about a foot in length and made of a whalebone wrapped in a strip of leather. I was, by and large, a well-behaved child, but I still fell foul of the rules and was caned on two occasions, once on the hand and once on the backside, with the ferula delivering instant, searing pain and stinging red welts that lasted through the night. In other words, the Jesuits were both pastoral and punitive figures, a combination familiar to anyone who's been in an abusive relationship.

I still believed in God back then. I was fearful, dutiful and compliant – unquestioningly accepting a regime of daily prayers and Mass every Sunday and holy day of obligation, the heady incense and the little Pavlovian bells that rang throughout the service inducing an almost hypnotic state in me. The chapel where we attended Mass was lined with realistically rendered images of the fourteen stations of the cross, Christ's final moments. Despite being too young to watch excessive violence or horror on television, I frequently found myself contemplating paintings of a man stumbling over rocky ground under the weight of a huge wooden cross, his head bleeding from the crown of thorns he was wearing, and then the same man nailed by his wrists and feet to the cross, blood gushing from his wounds. We were reminded at every turn that Christ died this agonising death for our sins, even though we were only children. The idea of suffering was reinforced in the liturgy, which was filled with mentions of pain, blood, sacrifice, flesh and death. At every Mass, we boys would receive communion from the very hands that had beaten us. Looking back in therapy, I saw it as indoctrination, overwhelming and disturbing in its delivery.

Inevitably, scrutinising that period of my life in therapy led to a moment of quiet rage. I could not believe that my parents left me in that place or sent me on to Ampleforth, with its own set of emotional challenges, later.

This is a common awakening for many clients, when they realise the damage that their parents may have caused, even unintentionally. For some, it is too much to forgive. They may choose to renegotiate the terms of the parental relationship or sever it altogether.

Thanks to Philip, I was able to be objective about mine. My father's career demanded a new posting every two years, meaning I would never have had the chance to settle in a local school. They were giving me consistency, as well as tapping into a generous boarding school allowance offered by the armed forces, which meant I could attend the kind of institution that would, at least theoretically, give me more advantages later in life.

What has subsequently been revealed about boarding schools – the damage they cause, the scandals that have engulfed many of them – was simply not known then. My mum and dad were doing what they thought was best, based on the information they had at the time.

This understanding stayed with me for decades. It felt like enough. Something I didn't need to question.

But our relationship with the past is constantly evolving. Experiences in the present can force us to revisit what happened years before, to seek fresh understanding, to reframe. And during my therapy sessions with Anna, this was exactly what happened to me.

CHAPTER 16

'Every person must choose how much truth he can stand.'
IRVIN YALOM

ANNA

For decades I despised and reacted physically to the word 'rape'. I couldn't say it, write it or even read it. To me, it was a dirty word and made me feel like a victim – which was something I didn't want to be. So, if I didn't say the word, write it, read it or even think it, I could pretend it didn't apply to me. I also hated the terms 'victim' and 'survivor'. I didn't want to be either of those things; I only wanted it to never have happened.

It was only a few sessions into our work when Paddy first used that word.

Unable to communicate verbally, I handed my phone to him and he read my fragmented memories of the first time it happened. I had a number of confusing questions, especially about how much responsibility I bore for the events.

'You're not to blame, Anna. This was something that happened to you. That was uninvited. You were raped.'

I recoiled at the word, fidgeting in my chair. My nose wrinkled with revulsion; my cheeks burnt with humiliation. He let the word settle between us. It was too late to take it back – the word that I had long avoided was suddenly out there.

'I know it's a hard word to hear,' he said softly. 'Is it OK if I use it?'

No, I hate that repugnant word, I don't want it near me. 'You can, but I don't want to,' I replied.

And from then on, he would always ask me before he used it and when it was too uncomfortable to hear, we'd use 'the "r" word' instead. It might seem silly that a four-letter word could evoke such a visceral reaction, but for me it represented so much more. It was a narrative I could not accept.

―――――――――― " " ――――――――――

PADDY

For the duration of our two years together, that word was always in the room. Like a ghoulish presence, it drifted in and out of focus, too ugly and painful for Anna to look at, let alone linger on. Seeking her permission before saying it out loud felt absolutely critical. It had to be her who decided what content she shared and at what pace. Her alone who shaped the narrative.

For me, a world of meaning is found in the words clients

choose, often at the expense of others with a similar definition, and how those words are expressed.

Some are spat out with disgust or venom. Some make clients stumble or stutter. Some words cause their voices to become timid whispers.

And then there are the words they dare not use, that hang, unsaid, in the room.

At times, when Anna spoke about her ordeals and downplayed or questioned what had happened, I wanted to shout the word out. But while this was frustrating, it was not my prerogative. And ultimately, it meant that when Anna was ready to own that word, she seized it with both hands and it became a weapon of huge potency and power.

ANNA

No one had listened. No one had noticed the pain or cared enough to ask. X had sent me the message that my wishes, and my body, weren't important. And when I'd tried to talk to friends, family and medical professionals, I was silenced or brushed aside. The truth was inconvenient and I was inconvenient. Eventually, I stopped talking, resorting to self-harm to deal with my pain instead.

Paddy, by contrast, wanted to listen. But by then, the habit of silence was deeply ingrained. I had so much to say, but I struggled to find the words. Almost twenty years of fear had kept me silent. I was scared of people's responses and reactions but absolutely terrified of X. And although his hand was no longer physically clasped over my mouth, the feeling had continued to linger. I couldn't acknowledge what had happened; it was too terrifying. I kept my mouth firmly shut.

Early in our work together, there was a moment when I was recounting part of the first incident. I was forcing myself to say it out loud, with Paddy as a witness. It was a kind of test to see if I could withstand it. Or to see whether I had healed at all.

But as I started to speak, I sounded distant and faint, and although I knew it was my voice, it was as if it belonged to someone else.

'I left the club. I was scared. I ran. I wasn't cold. There was a car. I bumped into X and... I... he...'

I trailed off, my thoughts tangled as the words stumbled over each other and I became ensnared in the images.

--- " " ---

PADDY

I could see Anna in front of me – her physical presence on the sofa – and yet I was losing her. As she descended deeper into her account of the incident, she seemed to disconnect from what she was saying. At first, it was like one of those news segments when an actor speaks the words of someone else and the delivery somehow lacks conviction and weight.

But then Anna took on a dream-like state. She was spaced out, like she'd taken drugs.

Anna was dissociating. We all do it. Think about those rote tasks – putting the bins out, commuting to work – when we sometimes switch off so we're not aware of the drudgery or monotony. In therapy, it's a coping mechanism, a form of pain management.

When clients re-experience unbearable trauma in counselling, they may feel their heart rate increase, sweat on their skin or an urge to run. That's one reaction. They may also experience a deadening of sensation, as if they're floating above the room and the therapist's voice is distant. Afterwards, they discover that they cannot remember the session.

Anna was in this latter state. In reliving her ordeals, she experienced an extreme level of threat in the room. By dissociating, she shut down and disconnected from a perceived danger.

The question for counsellors is when and how they bring the client back to the room.

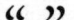

ANNA

'Anna?'

Paddy's voice seemed far away. I heard him, but it felt like he was on a different radio frequency and I was struggling to tune in. I wanted to communicate with him, but I couldn't speak. Or even move.

My brain sent a command to move my arm, my leg, *anything*, but it was as though the signal had got lost in the void between intention and execution, leaving me in a paralysed state – suspended between thought and action.

'Anna.'

I heard Paddy again. He seemed closer and a little louder than before. His voice acted as a lighthouse, guiding me back to safety amid a swirling sea fog. Reassuring and familiar.

―――――――――――――― " " ――――――――――――――

PADDY

By dissociating, Anna was in a softer, gentler place. It felt cruel, sadistic even, to pull her back into the room, where the very air swarmed with terrifying demons. But by telling her story in a dissociated state, she was not fully connecting to it and would not be able to process or integrate it. So, ultimately, no effective work could be done.

If clients persistently dissociate, therapists can bring them back in a number of ways – for example with a pre-agreed word or set of words or by nudging them to focus on an object in the room. They may also encourage them to press their feet to the floor, to feel the solidity of the ground beneath them.

That first time, I chose to invite her back by simply repeating her name, hoping that the soft tone of my voice would be enough to convince her that she was safe to return, that I wasn't going to force her to confront any monsters today.

I watched as a subtle change came over Anna. Her eyes became focused and her cheeks regained colour. Slowly, her shoulders dropped and she sank into the sofa as though she'd descended gently from the ceiling. Which, in a way, she had.

---- " " ----

ANNA

'I can't say it. I'm sorry. I feel like a failure. I really wanted to be able to say it.'

'Do you need to?'

'I don't know, I feel like I should be able to. Ages ago, I saw an article that said that once I'd processed everything, I'd be able to think about the events as I might a shopping list. I'd feel no emotion. I hoped I could, but I couldn't get past a few words. It's so fucking frustrating.'

Tears pricked my eyes. Paddy gave me a reassuring smile. One that conveyed solidarity and support. A smile that said, 'I understand.'

---- " " ----

PADDY

I doubted whether Anna would ever feel as indifferent about her rapes as she might do a shopping list. But it wasn't the moment to dash her hopes.

'I want to get you to a place where the events of the past are accommodated,' I said. 'Where you don't feel terror every time you revisit them. Right now, as you build your accounts here, it seems entirely understandable that you're overcome by such fierce emotions.'

Anna threw herself back on the couch, collapsing into the upholstery. 'I'm fed up with sitting on this sofa, week after week. I thought I was getting stronger, but I'm just so annoyed with myself for not being able to say it aloud.'

'I can really feel your frustration and impatience on this,' I said. 'Perhaps there's another way.'

Writing had always served Anna well in therapy: the accounts on her phone and the emails she sent between sessions that clarified or added depth and meaning to our conversations.

'I just wonder whether, in your determination to say out loud what happened, you've set yourself an almost masochistic task. It's just a thought, but perhaps writing the accounts might give you the distance you need?'

ANNA

Hearing Paddy's suggestion gave me a moment of reprieve. A chance to be kinder to myself and permission to take refuge from the relentless hot terror that accompanied the vocalisation of my memories. I hoped that writing would give me the opportunity to express myself without fear or judgement and find a voice that transcended the limitations of speech. While I knew that ultimately there would be power in the spoken word, I was happy that there was another way to approach my task. It felt safer, at least for now, and with Paddy's encouragement, I began to write.

CHAPTER 17

'Pain is important: how we evade it, how we succumb to it, how we deal with it, how we transcend it.'
AUDRE LORDE

ANNA

Throughout therapy, self-harm was a constant, silent companion, one that would provide relief in moments of upheaval or chaos.

I felt completely ashamed of self-harming. I would hide it from everyone – from the judgemental gaze of the world and from myself at times – cutting in areas that could be easily obscured. After I told Paddy about my clandestine activity early on in our work together, he told me something that I'll never forget.

'I spoke to Sue about our work last week.' Paddy paused, almost as if anticipating a similar reaction to the last time he'd broached this subject with me.

I smiled. 'It's OK, I'm not going to have a hissy fit again. What did she say?'

'I talked to her about your self-harming and Sue said, "Anna wouldn't do it if she didn't need to."'

I sat contemplating this for a moment, repeating the words in my head. *Anna wouldn't do it if she didn't need to.* Then something clicked into place. It was like someone finally understood that I didn't *want* to hurt myself, but it was, in fact, necessary. A tool for self-preservation. I felt a wave of acceptance engulf me. Of course, the self-judgement was much harder to tackle, but for now it felt as if there was no judgement in the room.

Having that acceptance was paramount as I began to write. From the brief account I'd shown Paddy on my phone in that first session, I began to draft a more comprehensive version of what I'd endured at the hands of X. It felt necessary for me to write every graphic detail, the numerous injuries I'd received, the spinning trees, the colour of the tiles on the floor, the burn of his stubble, the smell of his aftershave and the sensation of his breath on my neck. It felt as if the memories had shattered into thousands of pieces of glass and as they returned, I could feel every single one being painfully dragged back together. It was crucial to recount every detail correctly, and I'd become upset when there were shards of memories missing or I couldn't recall specific facts. If I couldn't remember what shirt X wore, or what dates the assaults happened on, it made my entire story a lie. And it made me question my own memories.

The details and chronology felt vital to me and it took time to place my regular flashbacks into the correct order. At first, this gave me an opportunity to see how much I was to blame. I was genuinely confused that Paddy didn't view my accounts in the same way. It was clear to me that there, on the page, lay my mistakes, my choices.

The horrific facts, that up until now had existed only in my head, began to feel less overwhelming as I shared them. The accounts were so sickening and violent that I couldn't imagine ever revealing them to my loved ones and although I always assured Paddy that he didn't have to read the graphic details, I was always grateful that he did. I needed someone to witness my pain and appreciate how frightening the events were. For the very first time, I wasn't alone.

As the silence began to lift and I found ways to express my story, there was terror. And while the act of writing was cathartic, the real healing and work was in sharing my pain and receiving the responses I needed and deserved.

From the first moment I told Paddy what had happened, albeit a brief version via the notes on my phone, he believed me. Unlike other people, he didn't ask me to prove it and he assured me that I bore no responsibility. And while every time I revisited the events he would respond with empathy and kindness, I found them difficult to receive. His compassion wasn't something I wanted or enjoyed, but Paddy was persistent, often annoyingly so.

Each time I revealed a little more information, sometimes with nauseatingly lurid details, I'd panic. Mostly about whether he'd believe me, whether he'd be angry at me or would think I was worthless. I always had an overwhelming feeling that I was somehow in trouble. That X would find out that I'd talked. Then my thoughts would swing the other way and I'd think that if Paddy did believe me, he'd conclude that I deserved it or, knowing the violence of the assaults, he'd make me report X, or blame or shame me, or even take X's side.

Even worse was the idea that he might pity me or say something nice. With the exception of my husband, 'nice' wasn't a reaction I was used to, and while I knew that these were completely irrational and unfounded fears, horrendously inconsiderate responses were much more familiar to me. But for every negative reaction I had received in the past, my heart had broken a little bit more and my defences hardened.

It had taken me such a long time to start to trust Paddy, but writing my story reminded me of how people typically treated me when I was vulnerable and I'd instantly regret sharing it with him. I knew I was repeating old patterns of opening up and shutting down, but protecting myself was crucial. I was acutely aware that I was projecting my past experiences onto Paddy, and he never gave me any reason to suspect he'd respond unkindly, but sharing my story always scared me and made me want to retreat and push him away.

I hadn't been able to stop myself from being harmed in the past, but I was doing everything I could to stop it happening now. At the same time, I *knew* that I had to let Paddy in so he could help me. I *knew* I needed to be vulnerable and try to accept his kindness, but I didn't know how. It was easier and a far more familiar pattern if Paddy could be angry with me.

So, we had reached a point where I'd entrusted him with my story, my truth, my everything and if he reacted as I feared he might, I was sure the experience would break me. This was a critical moment.

'I've finished writing my account.' I'd provided Paddy with what I thought were complete memories of the events, but my instincts told me there was always something else missing; something I couldn't quite access, a faint outline that teased my mind while the details remained elusive. Frustratingly so. This time I felt sure that my account was as complete as it ever would be, and even if there were details missing, I didn't care.

'Would you like me to read it?' Paddy asked.

I twisted on the couch and wrinkled my nose in disgust. By this point, I had a good understanding of my behavioural patterns and although, logically, I knew that he would respond with his usual consideration, I was very aware of the ball of fear and dread churning in my stomach and how my cheeks flushed with shame. I wondered if it would help to share what I was feeling.

'It's the usual paradox of desperately not wanting anyone to know but needing to have it acknowledged at the same time. I can't decide if one outweighs the other.'

He gave me a knowing smile to suggest we'd been here before. 'So, what are the benefits?'

'I feel like I need my story to be heard. To have a voice finally, I think, is important,' I said, sitting a little taller. 'I think I trust you enough, but I also feel very, very uncertain and distrustful of pretty much everyone. I've put up a lot of my walls again and I'm very wary of letting anyone back in. I don't want to bare my soul only to have it ripped to shreds.'

'I'd like to invite you to remember the things I've said and how I have reacted in the past when you have shared with me.'

'You'll say it wasn't my fault, but then you'll read it and you'll know that it was!'

'It wasn't your fault, Anna.' He must have repeated this line hundreds of times and although I always heard him, I never truly believed it.

'Can I email it to you to read before the next session? I couldn't bear for you to read it aloud.'

'Of course.'

―――――――――――― " " ――――――――――――

PADDY

Whenever Anna revealed details of her rapes, there was always an emotional hangover. She emailed after our sessions so many times, revealing more shame and embarrassment about giving so much away.

To give a sense of how deeply affected she was, here's an email from me, in which I address a series of fears she'd expressed after sending me her full account of both traumas.

Hi Anna,

Thank you for sending me this, which I will read before our next session. I know that every time you reveal more, it is terrifying. I just wanted to reassure you that my acceptance remains unchanged. But just in case you're still worrying – which I'm sure you will be – I've responded to each of the bullet points in your email.

I hope this helps a little. I understand your trust in others is fragile. But please know that I remain deeply committed to supporting you. We have come so far in counselling. Let's continue together and help you find resolution, closure and peace.

- *I worry that you won't believe me.* I still believe you and always have, Anna.
- *If you think something happened, I fear that you will blame me for being drunk or wearing certain clothes or for not being clear enough about what I didn't want. Or think it was a grey area.* Something did happen. You were attacked and raped. It doesn't matter what you wore or how much you had drunk. It was not a grey area. And it was never your fault.
- *If you know the details, you will certainly think even more badly of me (think I'm a slut).* I will never think badly of you. This was visited on you. You did not make it happen.
- *You will think I'm even more fucked up than you thought.* You are not fucked up. You are traumatised. For good reason.
- *You will take X's side.* That will never happen.
- *You will shame me.* I will not.

- *You will react in the same way as all the other people in my life have when I've shared it. And you will use what happened to hurt me somehow.* I will not. My only concern is your well-being. And I will continue to be here, whatever you share.
- *You will think I'm dramatic, hyperbolic, ridiculous, attention-seeking.* I do not think you've ever been those things. You deserve to be heard, believed and validated.
- *You will hate me. Loathe me as much as I loathe myself at times. Hate me as much as others have.* I continue to think incredibly highly of you – as a mother, human being and client, who is working incredibly hard to process her trauma.
- *You will think I deserved it, if you believe me at all.* As I said, I have always believed you. You never deserved any of this. You deserved happiness and a future and that was taken from you in the cruellest way possible.
- *You will stop helping me. I won't be worthy of help.* I remain 100 per cent committed to helping you.
- *You will see me as a victim. Label me. Think I'm weak, cowardly, pathetic.* Never.
- *You will pity me.* Never.
- *You will blame me for not running away.* Never.
- *You will blame me for not fighting.* Never.
- *You will blame me for not reporting X.* Never.
- *You will think I've contradicted myself somehow and therefore I am a liar.* You have never contradicted yourself in your accounts.
- *You will realise what a horrible, vile person I really am.* You

are none of those things. You're kind, considerate and compassionate.
- *I will be so afraid of the bad reactions, I'll push you away or self-sabotage.* You may do this, but I'll still be here.

--- " " ---

ANNA

When I finally emailed Paddy my full version of events, I was terrified. I'd tried to work out why I was so scared and drew up a list of what I knew were irrational fears. When Paddy responded, addressing my concerns, the weight of my worries lightened. His message spoke volumes – that no matter what I shared with him, his acceptance of me would remain constant. I was valued for who I was and not what experiences I had survived. I knew that he would be there to support me and whenever my inner critic echoed loudly with other people's hateful messages, I tried to remember Paddy's reassuring words.

--- " " ---

PADDY

I imagine there are counsellors who'd read this and conclude that my response was excessive. That by offering Anna these assurances, I was encouraging dependency and helplessness.

Worse, that I was rescuing her, trying to soothe Anna's discomfort rather than help her move through it.

I believe my response was necessary. Anna was able to hear my words, and the persistent message that I believed her, and come back with renewed strength. She understood at a core level that resolution lay in examining her pain, not swerving it.

For Anna, accuracy was everything. It was incredibly important to her to pin down the chronology and accurate details in her accounts.

Her painstaking approach reminded me of a defence lawyer preparing for trial.

'It's as if you're assembling evidence that's going to be presented in court,' I said one day. 'And if you get one element wrong, you'll be torn to shreds by some vicious Rottweiler of a prosecution barrister.'

Anna shrugged, as if this was hardly surprising. She'd been doubted and disbelieved by so many professionals and so-called friends. Why would she not be guarded and paranoid?

'In reality,' I continued, 'the only prosecution lawyer is the one inside your head.'

'Perhaps.'

I knew she understood what I meant, but she was not ready to accept it. It struck me that she was far more comfortable staying in that place of hypervigilance, where she remained ready to tear her account to pieces. Believing otherwise – accepting the entire truth of what she'd written – meant knowing that someone had done something truly horrifying to her. And if she wasn't to blame, and he was, a monster emerged fully formed in her head.

I'm a confident therapist, but as the weight of her experience sank in, I had a moment of crippling self-doubt. I'd seen clients with a history of trauma before, but I'd encountered nothing on this scale – in particular, the sustained and brutal nature of the second rape. I began to worry that I was hopelessly out of my depth.

I took my concern to my supervisor. Sue told me about a book called *Unshame* by Carolyn Spring, a trauma survivor and educator. It's about her journey to recovery and how she underwent therapy after the historic trauma that she'd successfully 'unremembered' for years manifested itself in a breakdown and dissociative identity disorder. The therapist who proved so pivotal in her recovery, and with whom Spring spent the better part of a decade, was a trainee.

Sue's point was that I didn't need a master's degree in trauma studies to help Anna. Spring's recovery was proof that, while experience is useful, it's the power and energy of the therapeutic relationship that is the most effective agent of change.

Did Anna and I have that? I had to hope we did.

A positive sign came not long afterwards, when Anna spoke about a dream that suggested we had created an alliance in therapy and that she was beginning, tentatively, to look to the future with more hope.

She described a scene in which there were two versions of her. There was an Anna standing on a black shingle beach, another on a soft, flower-covered cliff above the shore. The sea was pink and a storm was approaching; the sky was filled with large black clouds. She described feeling envious of the Anna standing on the cliff, who was 'free', but she also remembered thinking that the sea and sky were beautiful.

We discussed Anna's dream and took from it that she was able to occupy two places: one in which she faced the storm head on, another where she viewed it from a distance, amid the comfort of the flowers on the cliff. Looking at the dream together, it felt as if Anna knew a part of her had to face the storm head on. She was waiting for the oncoming tempest, the sea almost tinged with blood, while standing on black shingle that had once been lava due to a violent eruption. There was violence ahead and violence underfoot. The other part of her could remain at a safe distance, in a gentler environment. She might not have totally given me her trust, but she was beginning to recognise that counselling could be not only a place in which she could face her darkest memories but also a place to which she could safely retreat. I also wondered whether the beauty she saw in the storm was her acknowledging that one day, the truth would be liberating.

CHAPTER 18

PADDY

Therapists cannot afford to lose themselves in their clients' pain. What use are we to them if we're sobbing with sadness or numb with shock? A degree of separation is vital as we walk with them, a calm and trusted travelling companion on their therapeutic journey.

Separation is one thing. Detachment another. Given the explicit and disturbing nature of Anna's account, which I reread every time she revised or added to the content, it struck me that my reactions were unusually muted. During the sessions, I felt anger and sorrow about what had happened to her, but afterwards I found I could return to my life as if the past fifty minutes had barely touched me. On the one hand, it was useful. My work as a therapist remained in the counselling room. On the other, it felt a bit peculiar, like a switch was flipped inside my head every time and I ceased to feel.

One evening, I went to a lecture given by a British human rights lawyer who had worked to secure the release of dozens of innocent Guantanamo detainees. He was a charming and articulate speaker, his talk peppered with a dry wit that softened the impact of his tales of injustice, incarceration and torture. Towards the end, the lawyer recounted what I thought was a fascinating story. He and his team were at the prison recording a captive's particularly harrowing account of rendition and torture in preparation for an appeal. As the man revealed details of his experience of waterboarding, members of the legal team became distressed and, one by one, excused themselves until it was just the lawyer in the room. Later, when the team asked him how he had managed to endure the story, he realised that he was somehow resistant to the horrors because, like the detainee, he had also been waterboarded. His experience, he wryly revealed, was not at the hands of the CIA but courtesy of bullies at his boarding school, who had bog-washed him.

I suspect that bog-washing occurs in any institution where boys or men are cooped up together, but I know from Ampleforth and from friends who attended similar establishments that it was adopted with particular relish by British public schools. Bog-washing is when a victim's head is pushed down into a toilet bowl and held there while it is flushed, sometimes repeatedly. It is humiliating and terrifying. The victim begins to run out of oxygen and becomes convinced they're going to drown, which induces panic. They struggle against the hand that's pressing on their head, but because they're on their knees and most likely held down by someone older and stronger, they're powerless. Unlike the CIA's variation, where obtaining intelligence was the goal, bog-washing is only ever about sport and power. I hope to God it's not still practised today.

For many people who've survived trauma, encountering a stressor that mimics their original experience can be damaging, even devastating in some cases. It might be a smell or sound, a particular space, the light, an image, a person or event. It can be small, seemingly inconsequential, or something more dramatic. But if it's familiar enough, it can induce the symptoms of post-traumatic stress disorder (PTSD) – the anxiety, the flashbacks and nightmares, the intensely uncomfortable sensation of hypervigilance. At one point in her therapy, Anna had been triggered by a song playing on her car radio, with cruel irony, minutes before she arrived for a session.

In the lawyer's story, the detainee's account of waterboarding was so harrowing that it drove the other members of his team from the room. But he stayed till the bitter end. I'm not suggesting he should have been retraumatised by it, but to not be even slightly affected when the rest of his team had to exit the room, and to assume that his personal experience of something akin to waterboarding had somehow inured him to such an upsetting recollection, spoke of a profound detachment.

Following his lecture, I found myself thinking about my reactions to Anna's traumatic accounts.

I revisited my therapy with Philip, remembering something that at the time seemed inconsequential but now stuck out. I had processed a decade of boarding school experiences and yet I couldn't remember crying even once during the four years I was in psychoanalysis. Even the rage I felt was dialled down. There was no raised voice or gathering pulse. It was as if the desire to be polite and well-mannered trumped the need to express emotions. So, despite the work I put in, my feelings were muted, flickering like a gas hob on a low flame.

Years later, I read about the sexual abuse at Ampleforth and my emotional response, beyond my initial horror, soon dimmed.

I wondered whether that lawyer and I were the same creatures. As a child, I'd realised, at an unconscious level, that if I switched off my feelings, I couldn't be hurt.

Emotional cauterisation brings with it a thickening of the skin. It stops things getting through.

By the time I met Anna, I'd been practising for over a decade. I had thousands of client hours under my belt. I was an experienced therapist who'd regularly tapped into supervision to question, challenge and adapt my client work. But I felt like something was missing. My reactions to traumatic content simply weren't human. Possibly, they weren't even healthy.

I sensed that my clients would have been blissfully unaware. I'm confident that in sessions, they experienced me as compassionate. But I became convinced that if I didn't find a way to absorb and process emotional events, rather than brush them off like I was coated in Teflon, a part of me was in danger of calcifying.

CHAPTER 19

ANNA

Like Paddy, by the time I entered therapy I'd had decades of suppressing my emotions – switching them off or being unable to really look at them. And when I began to open Pandora's box and take the journey with Paddy, every step forwards involved reliving past horrors. He often spoke about a pendulum swinging in therapy and, at times, it felt like it was swinging between catharsis and torment. I also swung between a need for self-care and self-destruction or self-harm.

***

I sat on the couch, pulling a cushion onto my lap. My eyes fell upon the door, even though I'd only just walked through it. Paddy followed my gaze.

'Not keen on being here today?'

'Sorry. It's been a rough week.'

'Do you want to tell me about it?'

'I don't know where to start,' I sighed. 'It's just not fair.'

'What's not fair, Anna?'

'That I have to be here.'

'But you keep turning up.'

Silence.

'It was around this time of year', I said finally, 'that *it* happened.'

'It?'

'The first time,' I replied. 'I thought, or maybe stupidly hoped, that because I have been here for so long, it wouldn't affect me.'

Exasperated, I threw my hands up and inadvertently exposed my forearm with its two fresh cuts. I froze in absolute terror before a different kind of discomfort took hold of me. A warmth spread like wildfire, creeping across my chest and cheeks, turning them crimson. The awareness of being exposed and vulnerable was accompanied by a fear deep in the pit of my stomach. The urge to retreat and hide was overwhelming and I buried my head in my hands, covering my eyes.

'It's OK, Anna.' His voice was calm and quiet, as if speaking to a frightened child.

'But it's not,' I cried from behind my hands. 'You weren't supposed to see that. It's private.'

'Can you bear to talk about it?'

I forced myself to meet his eye, trying to find strength in the face of embarrassment. I nodded, hugging the cushion a little tighter.

'Do you want to tell me what happened?'

No, Paddy, I fucking don't. You've just witnessed the extent of my pain in its rawest form.

'I got upset last night. I think it was the anniversary of *it* – but I don't know the exact date.'

'And you ended up self-harming?'

No shit, Sherlock. I pulled my sleeves down over my hands and nodded.

'Can you remember what was happening for you just before?'

'Everything was building up inside. Disgust, shame. I felt like I needed to purge *him* from my body. I was angry, I think. And sad. It built and built until it reached a crescendo. I couldn't bear it any more and I—'

'Cut?'

'Yeah. For a few seconds, everything was calm. My thoughts were quiet; I had focus again.'

'It brought a degree of peace and clarity?'

'Yes, but then the realisation of what I had done sunk in. How would I hide it? Why was I so stupid? I hate doing it.'

'It served a purpose.'

'I suppose. But the way it makes me feel afterwards isn't worth it.'

'How does it make you feel afterwards?' he asked.

'Full of shame – which is stupid, because I am already ashamed. Regretful. Disappointed in myself. Weak because I can't control the urge. In pain, physically.'

'So, a barrage of self-critical messages.'

'Yes. I'm also terrified of the consequences – of people

seeing or finding out. Having to make up scenarios about how I became injured – like our pet rabbit scratching me – in case someone does see, and then feeling shit that I've made up a lie.'

'An exhausting process of covering up what you've done.'

'Exactly. And when you saw my arm today, I felt like I'd been caught out. I knew there was no point in lying to you. I also felt like I was in trouble.'

'You know what I'm going to say—'

'That I'm not. I logically know that. But I'm convinced you think it's disgusting. That I'm disgusting. That you might have sympathy for me being hurt by X, but how could you have sympathy for someone hurting themselves? But maybe that's a projection of how *I* feel about it.'

'And is that how you feel about it?'

'I suppose so. And I hate the thought that you might think that I do it for attention. That perhaps I showed you my arm on purpose. That I'm childish and attention-seeking.'

'I don't think that, Anna. I know how you detest it. And I know that you always hide it well. I'm more concerned that you cut in a visible place. I know from what you've said before that you would only ever harm yourself in an area that could be seen if you were in deep distress.'

I couldn't meet his eye. I saw the truth there.

'You feel terrible,' he continued, 'and yet every time there's still a powerful need. Do you have a sense of what that need might be?'

I stopped fidgeting and tried to think. But it was as if each thought was a note hinting at the melody of a half-composed song, like the semblance of something tantalisingly close, yet frustratingly out of reach. I wanted to run and leave the room again and I could feel myself drifting away.

'Anna?'

I forced myself back into my body, tensing the muscles in my legs. Suddenly, I became aware of pain pulsing along my forearm, demanding my attention. It helped.

'Maybe part of it is about control?' I offered.

'In what way?'

'That it's my body and I get to choose who hurts it? I don't know, perhaps that doesn't make sense.'

'The way that you were introduced to self-harm certainly wasn't in your control.'

'No, it wasn't. But the people who hurt me have long gone and for some reason I'm now the one hurting myself.'

'Perhaps being in pain is familiar?'

'It's another bloody paradox – the actions I'm taking to alleviate my suffering are the very things perpetuating it.'

'Fighting pain with pain?'

'Exactly. But how else do you fight pain?'

'With compassion, Anna.'

CHAPTER 20

Bristol, July 2020

ANNA

As we leave the student halls and walk back through the now wide-open gates, I feel enraged at the university's complacent approach to security. But I also know, from reading endless statistics, that the majority of rapes are perpetrated by acquaintances of the victim. And I finally understand, in that moment, that no amount of security would have protected me or prevented me from being raped by someone I trusted.

The smouldering anger that has been quietly bubbling away since we entered the city has become volcanic, threatening to explode. I breathe in and another lengthy sigh escapes my lips.

" "

PADDY

We're on the move again. Crossing the city to our next destination, a bar which Anna visited on the night of her first rape. The streets around the halls are mercifully quiet, but I spot busier roads ahead. Cars buzz by and the pavements are beginning to fill a little.

To the side of me, Anna performs a small ritual, as if shrugging off bad vibes. She turns to me and smiles. It's a reassuring sign. We still have work to do, but she appears to be in a secure place.

———————— " " ————————

ANNA

I walk with a sense of purpose. I feel taller somehow. Prouder, perhaps.

However, much like my drunken rollerblading friend who'd had a sudden flash of panic just before she fell, my bravery flickers as we reach a populated area. I begin feeling hypervigilant, increasing my speed, avoiding as many people as I can. Luckily, Covid helps me out and pedestrians seem just as keen to avoid us.

As we weave our way through scaffolding blocking the pavement, I see our next destination up ahead. I recognise the bar straight away. The name has changed, of course, and the neighbouring buildings have been demolished and rebuilt, but there's no mistaking it. An imposing three-floor red-brick building with meandering vines creeping across the lower levels. It's both impressive and terrifying. I recognise the area outside where I'd queue up with my friends to get in, talking to the bouncers to distract us from the bitter cold wind that whipped around the sides of the building. However, the only vivid memories I have of this bar, of both its interior and its exterior, are from that night. And shrouded in darkness. They are memories of feeling scared and confused. But it looks so normal in the daylight. Unassuming. And I feel slightly silly for being scared of a building. We both stand there in silence, the air charged.

'How do you feel?' Paddy asks.

'Stupid,' I blurt out without thinking. My self-blame resurfacing.

I realise it's probably the third time I've said this. I'm irritated that I've said it so many times because I now know that I'll be challenged on it. And, of course, Paddy picks up on it immediately.

He turns to look at me. 'Stupid?'

That simple, effective, yet bloody annoying therapist trick of repeating a client's words back to them.

I want to scream, '*I feel stupid! Like it's all my fault and I'm to blame! Stupid for getting drunk, for wearing what I wore, for leaving a nightclub alone, for everything. Everything. I even feel stupid for feeling stupid.*'

But I know these are emotions that I'm not supposed to feel. We've covered this in therapy. A lot. They're emotions that are supposed to belong to someone else. But stupid seems to cover everything, in that moment anyway.

I don't scream out; I don't even open my mouth. Once again,shame silences me.

'Yeah,' I manage to mumble eventually, the new self-compassion I found at the flats disappearing.

We stand across the street directly opposite the bar, silently observing. I don't need Paddy to say or do anything. Just knowing I'm not alone is enough in this moment. Time seems to stop yet continues around me. I'm frozen to the spot, caught somewhere between the past and the present. A couple passes us, their arms filled with shopping bags; a taxi rank operates outside. Life carries on for the rest of the world as they go about their daily routines. Everything just seems so... normal.

———————— " " ————————

PADDY

As we pause opposite the bar, there's a flash of blue light and a sudden burst of siren which makes us both jump. To our left, a police car has pulled over and two officers step out wearing face masks. They approach a homeless man sprawled on the pavement. We turn and stare – it's impossible not to – but

I'm also aware that neither of us will be able to concentrate until this commotion is over. It's an unexpected moment we have perhaps not prepared for specifically but we at least anticipated. Next, an ambulance arrives and the man is carefully helped into the rear by paramedics. Ordinarily, this would be a sad but fairly standard incident in a city centre. But in the aftermath of a pandemic, it appears utterly dreamlike and unsettling. We're all still so wary of other humans, yet here on the pavement, there's a tight dance of five people.

Pandemic or not, it's a blast of noise and unhappy drama, and I'm hoping it hasn't disturbed Anna as she contemplates the bar. As the vehicles move off, I glance at her. She nods back. The bubble appears to be intact.

———————————— " " ————————————

ANNA

I'm inwardly focused, viewing the outside world through a frosted windowpane, when the sudden shrill sound of a siren cuts through the haze. I'm jolted back to the present as police officers and paramedics attend to a man who has collapsed along the street. Even though I'm fixated on my mission, it's hard to retain a sense of normality, as the boundaries between reality and the absurd become blurred.

A barman comes out of the pub, opens the gates and places an A-board outside. I look at Paddy.

'Do you want to go inside?' he asks. 'It seems like a sign.'

I hadn't anticipated this possibility and it isn't contained in the four-page document that I wrote in an attempt to control and plan for every eventuality. Time catches up with me with a rush of momentum and propels me into the present. I take a deep breath and smile as I think of the friends who told me I'd end up in a pub on this trip. I have to trust that Paddy can support me through this.

'Yes,' I say with certainty.

As we cautiously step inside, I'm grateful that it's completely empty. The barman approaches us, asks if we want to eat and begins to tell us about the specials available. Thankfully, Paddy politely interrupts him and declines. I just want the man to go away so I can get out of here as soon as possible.

The interior is unrecognisable and it feels comforting to see that things have changed. They've moved on. And it's as if I can physically feel an internal shift. The vague memories of where the dance floor and the bar used to be are replaced with new images that seem more vivid and powerful.

———————— " " ————————

PADDY

It's the shortest of visits. Unlike at the flats, we cannot linger in a bar without ordering something and although no one says anything, it's obvious that neither of us wants the interruption that eating will bring.

As we emerge back out into the sunshine, I glance at Anna. I can't read the expression on her face.

———————————— " " ————————————

ANNA

'How are you doing?' Paddy asks.

'I don't know. Sorry, I know that's not helpful. I feel... different.'

'Different?'

'Good different. Like things have been reordered,' I ramble. 'The bar is in a different place and the dance floor isn't there any more.'

'Interesting. And how has that left you feeling?'

'I think... new? Refreshed?' I try out a few words before settling on 'lighter'.

But, as I step out onto the street, I hear a car horn in the distance and it triggers a brief flashback of a taxi braking and beeping its horn as I ran out into the road on *that night*. The power I felt after visiting the club is torn away in an instant. I become hyperfocused and walk off quickly, pointing out familiar landmarks. It feels crucial to me that I can prove to my therapist, and to myself, somehow, that the events really took place. Look, there are the flats I described to you, there's the nightclub that I left, this is the route home that I took. You see? I wasn't making it up.

I worry that if I've misremembered one small detail then I cannot trust any of my memories. But there is an internal sense of relief, perhaps even smugness – that things *are* how I remembered and described them. And perhaps now that Paddy has witnessed the images I'd meticulously described over and over again, he will finally believe me.

The relief doesn't last long and it's replaced by the absolute horror that, actually, things are exactly how I have remembered. Images that previously occupied the edges of my mind, blurred like bokeh, are now brought into clear focus and are indisputable. They are now the cornerstones of my understanding, leaving me with no room for an alternative reality.

CHAPTER 21

'Anger is better. There is a sense of being in anger. A reality and presence. An awareness of worth. It is a lovely surging.'
Toni Morrison, The Bluest Eye

ANNA

The next time I sat on Paddy's couch, the atmosphere was different from the usual calm that he provided.

We made brief small talk about the weather and his dog, but I felt the presence of unsaid words. I wasn't sure if Paddy had read the account that I emailed him before the session. I tried to remember what he'd written, when he'd reassured me of his unwavering acceptance. Not knowing how to approach the subject, I waited patiently and was thankful when Paddy finally addressed the unspoken.

'I've read it,' he stated simply.

Embarrassment flooded over me and my gaze immediately fell to the floor. My knee began vigorously bouncing up and down and tears brimmed at my eyelids, like water at the edge of a dam, threatening to overspill. I was transported back to those early sessions, when I was unable to meet his eye. *Stop it. You can do this. Put your head up. He said it wouldn't change how he sees you. Believe him.*

I swallowed. Hard. The tears retreated as I lifted my head up and looked at him. And, for the very first time, I saw my pain reflected in his face. I was confused and unsettled – this wasn't the reaction I was used to. But suddenly, his expression turned to anger – a much more familiar response.

His cheeks were flushed and his fists began to clench. 'I'm furious!' he exclaimed.

I felt fear gripping me. It was so familiar, yet always so unwanted.

'At me?' *Shit, maybe I shouldn't have told him.*

'No, of course not, Anna,' he said, still seething. 'He's a fucking monster.'

---- " " ----

PADDY

I'd felt anger before. But not like this.

Usually, it passed after reading her accounts, like skin swiftly healing over a cut. But on this occasion, the wound continued to feel fresh and sharp, as if salt were being sprinkled over it.

There was nothing about this account that changed the facts, but Anna had added new details to the version she'd emailed. She always wrote with such clarity, so viscerally, and this time the images stuck in my head.

It wasn't just what she'd written about how X had acted, although that was enraging enough.

It was, I see now, what I was carrying inside me.

It was a fury I'd never fully acknowledged, let alone expressed.

———————— " " ————————

ANNA

Paddy's reaction was one I'd never encountered in the past from others. Disbelief, blame and occasionally pity, and so much anger directed towards me, but never at X. Paddy softened and his rage dissipated as quickly as it had arisen, as if he was painfully aware of my discomfort.

———————— " " ————————

PADDY

I was surprised, even shocked at the words I'd used to describe X. At the force with which I'd uttered them.

'Fucking monster' wasn't my usual therapeutic turn of

phrase. In fact, it didn't sound like something I'd ever utter in a session.

My heart was galloping and my cheeks felt hot. I worried that Anna might have noticed. She needed me to be her calm companion not an angry man, in this of all places.

I could not let that happen or let my anger contaminate the session, so I did what I'd encouraged Anna to do so many times in the past. I breathed in deeply, then exhaled slowly.

I felt a degree of calm return. Across the room, Anna looked a little bewildered, as if she was thrown by what I'd said or the strength of my delivery.

The session progressed, but given how much she'd revealed – more than ever before – and my unexpected reaction, it felt important to me to end the hour with a more composed message. It was one she'd heard from me too many times to count, but I felt it always bore repeating.

'I will say it again because it can never be said enough. There is not one single part of this that you either caused or deserved. You bear no responsibility. It doesn't matter what you were wearing or how much you had drunk. Nobody has the right to do what X did. This was inflicted on you by a brutal man who betrayed your friendship and trust in the cruellest way imaginable.'

I wasn't sure whether she'd heard me any more clearly today than in the past. But for some reason, I heard myself. The words seemed to ripple through me.

―――――――――― " " ――――――――――

ANNA

As usual, I heard Paddy but couldn't agree with him.

The session left me with a number of confusing thoughts. I had been stuck in my rigid pattern of self-blame, downplaying the events that had happened and remaining stoic. *For twenty years*. Was it possible that there was an alternative? Why was Paddy so bothered about something that 'may have happened' almost two decades ago? I didn't have any proof that the events had even occurred. Calling X a monster confused me further – was the incident really that bad? And if it was, had I been letting a monster roam free for the past twenty years?

———————————— " " ————————————

PADDY

I didn't fully understand it at the time, but Anna's account had a profound effect on me. Finally, I was able to express a rage that had been locked away for decades. Maybe it had been brewing for months. But it was as if her final account, so raw in its description of a man's brutal behaviour, had torn the lid from the bunker in my head.

I meant what I said about X. In my supervision, I'd even admitted to Sue that I'd fantasised about tracking him down and killing him. But behind my comment existed a wave of rage about other men. The men of God who stood in the pulpit on Sunday preaching to teenage boys about sins of the flesh and the sanctity of confession, who, under their saintly façade, were sexual abusers who destroyed their victims' childhoods and any hope of future happiness.

Not just those men but also the ones who had protected them and covered up their crimes. The authorities at the school who would have known for decades but never contacted the police, acting instead in self-interest and putting the reputation of the school and monastic community before the needs of the pupils, the very children they'd been entrusted to protect.

CHAPTER 22

ANNA

As I processed the session in the following days, Paddy's anger became hugely helpful. It enabled me to acknowledge that perhaps what had happened wasn't OK – that the events I'd downplayed *were* actually that bad.

I'd only ever experienced anger where it had been directed towards me. It felt frightening and overpowering. My past told me that anger was used to control, humiliate and intimidate. It could be used as a weapon and it felt punishing and destructive. Anger scared me, because I didn't want to be like the people who had hurt me. I'd always prided myself on not carrying hatred or anger. Despite what others had inflicted on me, I felt that I could keep my integrity by refusing to hate them or let them affect me, but this only resulted in a slow destruction from the inside.

Paddy attempted to show me that anger could be healthy, a valid emotion that I was entitled to.

For the very first time, I began to feel angry towards X.

However, after nearly twenty years of suppression, the results were not pretty.

***

Shortly after I had shared my full account with Paddy, a song came on the radio one evening, long after the children had been put to bed. It provoked such terror and a crippling physical response in me. Somehow, I'd always managed to avoid the song until now, diving across the room to turn it off as soon as I heard the familiar intro, but this time I forced myself to listen. As I sat cross-legged on my bedroom floor, memories of the friendship X and I once had came flooding back in a confusing mess of loss, nostalgia and all-encompassing fear. But, this time, there was also a new emotion. At first, just an irritation that X had ruined my enjoyment of music, and then a rising anger about this injustice – WHY ME?

As the song continued to play, I started to cry. It felt confusing. Unnatural. Scary, even. I'd always bottled up my pain and I didn't know how to deal with any emotion, let alone all of them crashing over me at once, so I berated and blamed myself for not knowing, for feeling confused, for crying and for everything.

Unwanted images entered my mind – X's hand clasped over my mouth, his forearm across my neck. Refusing to have yet another panic attack, I dredged from somewhere deep in my mind Paddy's advice to breathe out slowly. I could see X standing over me, laughing, and the past and present became entangled. Although rationally, I *knew* he wasn't with me, it felt like I was back in my flat as a student but also as if he was there in my family home. I became consumed with rage. Everything hurt and I needed to find a way to halt these raw and unwanted feelings. Making a tight fist, I pictured his face, and as the tears distorted my vision, I punched the rough and unforgiving brick wall in front of me.

I looked down, feeling no pain, only numbness and adrenaline rushing through my veins. Small continuous trails of crimson ran down from three badly grazed knuckles. I became swamped by shame, a much more familiar feeling.

I ran my hand under the freezing-cold tap, feeling undeserving of any warmth, and watched as the water turned pink and circled around the sink before disappearing. I felt detached and desensitised, as though I was watching someone else wash their blood away.

As I returned to the present, and the intense pain that accompanied it, I began to panic. Why on earth had I done that? How the hell would I be able to explain it? I fleetingly remembered we had a PTA school meeting the following evening and knew that I'd have to conceal it. Everyone would think I was crazy. I even had an appointment with Paddy in the morning and I definitely wouldn't be able to hide it there.

I winced as I tried to make a fist, simultaneously welcoming the pain, feeling fully deserving of it, yet frightened by my actions. No longer angry at X, I blamed myself entirely for the horrific events of the past and vowed to keep the anger turned inwards next time.

***

When Paddy opened the door the next morning, Lola

gleefully trotted out and I reached to stroke her before immediately remembering my knuckles and switching hands, terrified that my therapist might see. Thankfully, he didn't seem to notice.

'I've been reading,' I said proudly. Paddy had been encouraging me to rekindle my passions, both for self-care and as a route towards rediscovering a wider sense of self-identity. I'd picked up my camera again for the first time in years and when I'd taken my children to the library, I had grabbed a book for myself.

'*The Marsh King's Daughter*. I'm really enjoying it.' I was aware that I was avoiding what I needed to talk about.

Paddy was always happy to ease into a session with book talk, but on this occasion, he was quick to bring it back to me.

'I've read that book too,' he said. 'Is there anything in particular that you liked? Or perhaps resonated with?'

He's good. We both know that there are obvious parallels.

'There was a bit where she describes being in a "witness protection of her own design" – where she has to cut all ties with her old life to make the new one stick. It's like she couldn't let the two lives intersect.' I glanced at him, and although he didn't say anything, it felt as though he was rooting for me to make a connection.

'I think this is very similar to what happened with me,' I continued. 'In order to survive after being attacked, I had to bury everything. I made a different life with no reminders of the past. I'm paranoid about confidentiality and people finding out. Partly because I'm ashamed and feel weak for going to therapy but also because I don't want the two different parts of my life to overlap.'

--- " " ---

PADDY

'So, you saw something of yourself in her experience?'

Anna nodded.

The Marsh King's Daughter is a novel about a woman born and raised in an isolated cabin by her terrified mother and the brutal, psychopathic man who holds them both prisoner – her father. She later escapes and the life she goes on to lead reminded me so much of Anna. Despite her trauma, the woman shows incredible resilience – a fierce determination to survive and thrive, to bury the past until, out of the blue, she's forced to confront it.

The book is both a study of trauma and a tale of revenge. I wondered whether the protagonist's pain and rage had resonated.

'Was there anything else you connected with?'

It wasn't the most subtle of questions, but Anna was often happy to continue conversations about books and films. What began as small talk, a safe way to enter a session and warm up before the real work began, often drifted naturally into therapy, with Anna seeing her own experience mirrored on the page.

She responded in the most unexpected way.

ANNA

'I punched a wall last night,' I blurted out suddenly, unable to contain the secret any more.

My revelation left Paddy momentarily speechless, unable to hide his initial surprise and shock, but he quickly regained his composure.

'Did you hurt yourself?' he asked, with genuine concern.

'No,' I lied, as I held out my grazed and puffy hand.

'What type of wall was it?'

I frowned. *Walls are walls, aren't they?*

'Chipboard? Plasterboard? Concrete?'

'Oh, right, erm, brick.'

He winced and although I felt immediate relief at not having to hide it any further, I was deeply embarrassed. Ashamed that a 35-year-old mum of three had punched a wall in anger. I needed to divert the attention away from myself.

'Have you ever punched a wall?'

We both knew I was deflecting and I didn't really expect him to answer.

'I have, actually.'

I was genuinely surprised, and relieved, by his answer.

'What kind of wall was it?' I asked sarcastically.

'Not brick, thankfully.'

PADDY

A psychodynamic therapist might have responded to her question with, 'I'm interested to know why you feel the need to ask?' But if I'd come out with something like that, Anna would have raised an eyebrow, unable to conceal her annoyance at having her question met with another question. We were way beyond that place. The best of our work was always achieved when we were truly human with each other. So, before I'd even had a chance to think, I responded honestly. As the words slipped from my mouth, I was surprised at my candour, but at the same time I was confident I was making the right decision.

For a brief moment, I was back there. The exact reason I hit the wall escaped me – it was decades ago – but I clearly recalled the sudden rush of rage, my fist flying out. Knuckles smacked into plasterboard, which crunched and collapsed, and while that was infinitely less painful than the punch Anna had described, it still left me with a livid wound across my knuckles which took days to heal.

So, I knew what it was like to suddenly feel overwhelmed by fury, by the urge to destroy something, along with the red-hot sensation of pain to match or even swamp the rage inside. I liked to think my anger had been muted in the past, but there had been moments when it rose in me like a volcano. And perhaps the mortification of the scabbing injury on my hand and the hole in the wall – which I swiftly filled in and painted over – had been enough to convince me that anger wasn't something that a man like me did.

Men like me kept emotion under wraps. The rage as well as the tears.

Snapping out of my memory, I thought about my decision to respond truthfully. I hoped it would show that Anna did not need to feel shame.

———————————— " " ————————————

ANNA

I didn't press him for details, and I didn't need to know, but his confession made me feel less alone and less like an utter madwoman, although I suspected that the other mothers at the PTA meeting would disagree.

———————————— " " ————————————

PADDY

I wanted to encourage Anna to maintain that, albeit brief, connection to anger and injustice in a healthier way, without hurting herself. I imagined her like the protagonist in *The Marsh King's Daughter* and hoped her rage could be powerful if harnessed in a constructive way. I took another chance.

'If X was here, in the room with us now, what might you say to him?'

A frightened look unfurled across her face. 'I'd be too scared. Terrified, in fact.'

'OK, what if he can't hurt you or respond?'

'So, he's tied up and gagged?'

'Yes, why not?'

She looked uncomfortable, but I pressed on. 'Be as colourful with your language as you like.'

'Erm, I don't know. I guess I'd say, "You weren't very nice to me."'

'Go on.'

'Erm, I might tell him he's a wanker? Sorry, I don't know what to say,' she giggled nervously, evidently uncomfortable at expressing herself on this occasion.

Anna wasn't ready to say what she really thought. Remembering her email describing her anger at me and Sue, I suggested that she write a letter to X.

In therapy, letter writing can be an extremely powerful way to express emotions that prove difficult to voice. It can also offer a sense of distance.

Letters can be drafted and never sent. They can be kept as aides-memoire to revisit when a client needs to reconnect to a particular emotion. Or they can be destroyed (after securing their permission, I have often burnt clients' letters in the wood burner in front of them, a symbolic but powerful way to help sever the hold of a particular emotion or episode).

They can also be sent but only ever after a discussion with clients about what response they need and how best to manage the outcome – that they may receive something quite different or, indeed, nothing at all.

CHAPTER 23

ANNA

I looked fondly at Lola, who was stretched out between us. Her head resting on my foot, her tail on Paddy's Converse, connecting us both.

'I wrote a letter, as you suggested,' I said, handing him my phone.

'Do you want me to read it out loud?' *Not really.*

'Erm, yes, actually. I think it might help.'

I was unsure whether it would help or not, but I settled back into the couch pretending to be more relaxed than I felt.

He read, keeping his voice devoid of intonation or inflection, like he wanted the power of the words to speak for themselves.

To X,

We both know what happened and the pain you inflicted upon me. You took what you wanted and left me broken.

Shattered into pieces when I was already so fragile. I've tried to live and function as a normal person, but I was living a lie. A flashback of your face, your smell, even the sound of a group of people walking past me and laughing would cause a painful shard to resurface. A memory or even just a feeling of pure terror. The thought of your breath on my neck still fills me with dread and haunts my days.

I've finally met someone who is helping me to put myself back together, one tiny piece at a time. And it's fucking painful.

You took everything from me and made me into the person I am today. A weak shell of a woman filled with pain, anger, sadness and grief. Too scared to sleep at night, too scared to think during the day. At times, too scared to go anywhere in case a smell or a sight triggers a memory and I have a panic attack in public. Constantly exhausted because I'm always looking for any sort of threat.

The fact that you just calmly forced yourself on me that first time, as if you weren't doing anything wrong, confused me for years. Had you meant to r*** me? Had I given off the wrong signals? Was it actually r***? Had I actually said no? But when you put your hand over my mouth and your arm across my neck, you turned into something else. Months of therapy have made me realise that no amount of denial will undo the fact that you r**ed me. That you pushed aside my underwear and my wishes. Ignored my struggles beneath your body and my pleas to stop. I trusted you. With everything I had. You managed to keep me quiet that night by physical force and then ensured I would keep your secret by making me fear you. I wish I could have done something to stop you from returning a second time.

I thought I was safe with you after leaving the club. I don't think I'll ever be safe again. You can reach me in my dreams and any time I close my eyes. Your face, your smell, your taste, your unwanted touch – ingrained for ever into my memories.

―――――――――― " " ――――――――――

PADDY

Even though I tried to read the letter with a degree of neutrality in my voice, I felt the words vibrate through me. I wondered if the act of writing had helped Anna to connect more fully with her anger.

Attached to the letter was a photograph that she had taken of waves crashing on the beach during a storm. It represented the power of the natural world. A force that could destroy but also reshape.

―――――――――― " " ――――――――――

ANNA

Paddy took a long breath in and handed me back the phone.

'That's a powerful, angry letter, Anna. The truth so unequivocally spelt out. How was it to write?'

'I didn't want to do it initially, so I put it off for days. But then I had a dream about X – just a load of flashbacks – nothing to analyse.'

'I'm sorry.'

'It's fine. And although I was frightened when I woke up, I was also really pissed off.'

'Is that a new feeling after a dream like that?'

'Yes. It was confusing. I felt like self-harming, but I started to write the letter instead.'

'And did you feel any sense of release?'

'Well, I didn't self-harm. But it's just so hard to think that I didn't have any part in it.'

'You didn't. It wasn't your fault.'

'I don't know. When I wrote the letter, I wanted to place the blame on him and felt some anger. But now I've reverted back to thinking everything was my fault.'

— " " —

PADDY

The exercise hadn't brought about the profound change I'd hoped for, but it signalled that there had been progress. Anna had connected to her anger again. She had started to think, even if only momentarily, that she wasn't to blame. And even if she'd swung back the other way, it gave me hope that things were moving in the right direction.

CHAPTER 24

PADDY

About a year after the Independent Inquiry into Child Sexual Abuse published its findings on Ampleforth, I was invited to a lavish birthday bash thrown by an old friend from school.

I arrived late, parked in a field and made my way down a path lit by flaming torches to a terrace in front of his house. The event was already in full swing. There were around 200 guests, most of them dressed in outlandish costumes – a whiff of the party scene in *Saltburn* about the whole thing. Uniformed staff weaved their way through the throng, delivering cocktails or flutes of champagne, the warm summer air filled with notes of expensive perfume and the deafening roar of loud, posh, male voices. Below us, a huge marquee had been erected to host dinner and the dancing afterwards.

I grabbed a cocktail from a passing waiter and took a large gulp. This kind of occasion, which I very rarely go to, makes me nervous. Although I attended a fee-paying school, I'm not from a wealthy family. My parents were able to send me to Ampleforth because of the generous financial allowance provided by the army. What I'm trying to say is that I was educated with boys from very different families. I'm also not great in crowds, preferring smaller gatherings where individual voices are distinct and can be fully heard.

The party was a joint fiftieth and eighteenth and among the guests were many of my Ampleforth contemporaries and, as I soon discovered, their children, some of whom had also attended the school. At one point, I found myself chatting to a group of them – tall, handsome young men, about to embark on gap years or start university. They were charming, confident and optimistic, and it was hard not to be infected by their excitement about the future.

Later, I caught up with their fathers. Before long, the conversation turned to the revelations about the school, still fresh in everyone's minds although, as I was to learn, for very different reasons.

Recalling the evening now still feels surreal.

'It's ghastly,' said one.

'Just dreadful,' said another.

I assumed they were talking about the seriousness of the revelations and the horror perpetuated on boys as young as seven over several decades.

But no.

'I mean,' said the first one, 'there's a very real danger of the school closing if something isn't done.'

'They need to take control of the narrative,' said the other. 'If this goes on, no one will want to send their children there.'

With a creeping unease, it dawned on me that they were referring to public relations, about how to manipulate the story so that Ampleforth emerged in a more favourable light. I was speechless and in shock. I briefly zoned out as they began discussing the more positive attributes the school needed to highlight. I caught the occasional phrase: 'A-level results', 'Oxbridge entries', 'sporting achievements'.

Snapping back into the moment, I interjected, 'The report is damning. Do you not think this is the only story for now?'

'It's terrible what happened,' said the first man. 'But you can't condemn the whole school because of a few isolated incidents and a handful of individuals.'

'It's not a few isolated incidents,' I said. 'And there were many more—'

Our conversation was interrupted by another group of old boys arriving. There were hugs and back slaps and jokes were cracked. The mood changed in an instant.

There were more conversations about Ampleforth that evening. More former pupils who were disinclined to linger on the revelations. Men who were determined to focus on the positives and were committed to save a school that clearly meant more to them than confronting an ugly and inconvenient truth. They talked about their children's excellent exam results. The universities they were heading to. How their kids had been educated with the sons of old friends, like they were all one big happy family.

At no point did any of them express any sense of horror or anger. Instead, to a man, they sprang to the school's defence, like it was a helpless, cornered animal.

Given the scale of the abuse, there was a strong likelihood that boys we had known at school were victims. There was even the possibility that guests at the party had been abused. But if what I'd encountered so far that evening was anything to go by, it seemed that no one wanted to face the facts.

As the party meandered on, I became a little drunk, keen to numb the unsettling feelings I was experiencing. I met other guests, had conversations about other subjects. These diversions were a distraction, but there remained in my mind the lingering sensation that I was being gaslit.

Towards the end of the night, when other guests were either on the dance floor or outside enjoying the balmy air, I was wandering through the deserted dining area. The lights had been turned up and waiters milled around the room, clearing plates and glasses from the tables.

Across the marquee, I spotted someone I knew, the cousin of one of my peers, who'd been some years ahead of me at the school. He was in conversation with another man, although their body language suggested it was a fleeting exchange that was close to ending.

Your typical Ampleforth old boy works in the City or in a law firm. He might also serve in the army or sit as an MP or a peer (in both cases, most likely a Conservative). If he's the more curious or artistic type – although they were a minority – he might be a journalist, actor, musician or artist. What he doesn't tend to be is a psychotherapist or psychologist.

The man standing on the other side of the room was the only other old boy I knew of who had entered my profession. A well-regarded psychotherapist who'd worked in the NHS, Jock now practised as an organisational psychologist.

Standing in the middle of a party where everyone appeared to have blinkers on, I strongly hoped he might be willing to discuss what I knew to be true.

As the conversation across the room wound up, I approached him, introduced myself and asked if he minded having a brief chat.

We sat at a table while waiters quietly moved around us.

'This might seem strange,' I said, after a bit of small talk, 'but I feel like I'm in the *Twilight Zone*.'

Jock smiled. 'I think I may know what you're referring to.'

It turned out that he'd experienced exactly the same bizarre feeling.

'It's like I'm making the whole thing up,' I said. Saying this, I was briefly reminded of Anna, whose truth had been denied or dismissed so many times – by friends and professionals – that she shut down and later, when she finally began to speak, felt she had to constantly check and double-check the veracity of her account.

'You're not making it up,' Jock said, his face suddenly grave.

He went on to describe how his professional life had changed in the wake of the revelations.

'After the report was published,' he said, 'I began to be

contacted by old boys who'd been physically or sexually abused at Ampleforth. People have been hit really hard by this and they're desperate for support.'

He described men who'd previously had therapy, who'd found a way to live with what had happened to them, only to be retraumatised by the news. Others who had coped by burying their trauma deep had had the lid wrenched from their bunker. These men were in very raw, vulnerable places.

When I finally crawled into bed in the small hours, I felt a mixture of sadness and relief. It had been a comfort speaking to Jock. Now I knew for certain that I had been gaslit, perhaps not intentionally, by the old boys at the party – men who were determined, for reasons I had yet to understand, to deny the truth.

The sadness I felt was for those who'd been crushed by their childhood sexual abuse, an experience that, like rape, can spread its tentacles into every aspect of a person's life.

Adult survivors may carry an unbearable weight of guilt. They may believe they failed to stop the abuser and become convinced it was their fault. They may also feel guilty if at any time during the abuse they experienced pleasure, which can happen involuntarily as a biological response, despite the act being a violation. In numerous cases, that guilt morphs into shame. They may even conclude that they made the abuser think they wanted it. That they deserved it. That they're dirty and disgusting.

At a time when they should have felt safe and secure, the abused child instead feels threatened, terrified and violated;

their childhood shattered. It's little wonder that many adult survivors have problems with trust and struggle to form and sustain loving relationships. Child sexual abuse is often a person's first experience of sex. It can taint their sex life and prompt flashbacks and painful memories when they're intimate with others. Even if they do manage to form relationships, their past can still cruelly overshadow their lives.

An adult survivor may also have difficulties coping in the workplace and fail to achieve any form of financial stability. They may suffer with depression, anxiety, eating disorders or alcohol and drug addiction. They may even conclude that simply existing – carrying the weight of the past and all the feelings it elicits – is unbearable and choose to end their life.

After speaking to Jock, I no longer felt I was going mad. I knew the truth.

But the truth was accompanied by a terrible sadness. The report was a horrifying read, yet the unnamed victims had in some way become statistics. Jock had made them real. I pictured grown men unravelling, their already precarious lives crumbling, even as their fellow old boys laughed and joshed and denied their experiences.

I didn't sleep that night.

CHAPTER 25

ANNA

Like Paddy, I'd had many experiences of being gaslit by others – 'You're being dramatic', 'I don't believe anyone would do that!' And a cavalcade of other people's misogyny and myths: 'What did you expect, dressed like that?' and 'Why were you walking alone?' Until eventually, these messages were absorbed and became truths, shadowy whispers in my ear, internal biases, as if a silent puppeteer was pulling the strings of my thoughts and actions and guiding me down a path littered with misconceptions. And after years of being on the receiving end of doubt and dismissal, I began to gaslight myself.

From the very beginning of our work together, Paddy regularly challenged me on my rigid thinking.

'I'm so sorry that happened to you, Anna,' he said during one session. He liked to say this every now and then.

'It's not your fault,' I replied.

'Well, no. But I am sorry that those things happened to you.'

I shrugged my shoulders, dismissing his words and let them bounce off me with an air of indifference.

'You still don't believe me?' he said.

I turned to look out of the window, gazing at the beauty of the Devon landscape. Sam had taken the kids to the beach that morning and, more than anything, I wanted to be with them. *I want to leave. Why does X get to live his life happily ever after, while I'm stuck here week after week reliving the most painful times of my life?* I chewed my lip and crossed my arms. *Stop acting like a petulant child. Engage, he's trying to help you.*

I let out a sigh tinged with frustration – at the situation and at myself. I continued looking out of the window. 'I just know it was my fault.'

If Paddy was frustrated to have this conversation yet again, he didn't show it.

'What makes you think that, Anna?'

'I was drunk and I was wearing slutty clothes,' I stated matter-of-factly. I turned to face him.

'Slutty clothes?' he repeated, making direct eye contact and matching my tone, challenging me to think harder about those words.

I knew what he was trying to get me to say and I ignored him, pressing on. 'I found three articles last night that have shown that provocative dress can have an effect on the likelihood of sexual assault,' I said, handing him my phone with the abstracts I'd copied into a note.

'And what was the outcome of this one?' he asked, pointing to the first article.

'That the way a woman dresses is *sometimes* taken as a statement of her character. Of her vulnerability, of her, erm, *willingness* to have sex.'

'*Sometimes*. Sounds pretty flimsy. And this one?'

'That provocative dress *may* increase the chance of rape in *some* situations.'

Without looking at the third journal article, he handed me back my phone and exhaled, bringing a hand up to his temple. 'Anna, you've got two scientific degrees.'

He let the words linger, their inference clear. *How had I confused correlation and causation? Why had I trawled the internet to construct a poorly composed argument? Why was I so stupid?*

'I'm certain you can find anything on the internet that will prove your point. And I'm guessing you didn't search for pieces that opposed it?'

I dipped my head, 'No.'

He was silent for a few seconds, letting his words hover in the air and also, I suspected, formulating a measured response.

PADDY

'Anna, a woman is perfectly entitled to get drunk and wear what she wants without the threat of being raped. Nothing gives a man the right to do that.'

Anna looked at me, her lips pursed. Hearing my words but still unable to accept them.

'You are not to blame.'

'You would say that,' she said quietly, staring at my shoes, as she often did when the mirror she found in my face was too much. 'You're a therapist.'

'Yes, therapists will say a victim of rape is not to blame and, yes, I know you've heard me say it many times. But there's a reason I repeat the line and that's because it's true. Victims of rape are never to blame.'

She met my eye.

'Last year, the Met issued some advice to women in which they urged them not to wear headphones so they were alert to potential dangers.'

'I remember,' said Anna. She looked a bit smug, as if I'd just proved her point.

'Then you may also remember the backlash that followed.'

She seemed peeved, like I'd tripped her up.

I reached for my phone, where I'd saved a line that I wanted to read to Anna.

'A campaigner for victims of sexual violence came back with this,' I said. '"Headphones don't rape women, nor do skirts, or dark streets, or clubs, or alcohol, or parties, or sleepovers, or school uniforms."'

Anna was silent. Unable to provide a retort but unwilling to acknowledge the truth. 'Rapists rape, Anna. So, yes, as your therapist, I will repeat myself till I'm blue in the face and you're bored sick of hearing me. You are not to blame. X is a violent rapist. The blame lies squarely with him.'

" "

ANNA

Something inside me shifted slightly as I realised he had a point. However, I was unable, or perhaps reluctant, to extend his logic to my situation and I was ready to argue with him and prove that it didn't apply to me. I pushed on, but the rage that propelled my desire to debate had dissipated.

'I remember reading about an exhibition earlier this year called "What Were You Wearing?"' I said. 'It showed examples of clothes people were wearing when they were attacked. I *know* it doesn't matter what you wear – and the painful images of children's clothes made this extremely clear – but I honestly feel like in my case it did.'

My voice had become higher, cracking slightly as I tried to explain myself. I paused, teetering on the brink of vulnerability and a realisation that I was losing the argument.

'And what makes your situation different?' His voice was now less challenging.

Tears began to form and the veil between my internal world and outward expression became paper thin. A hard lump formed in my throat, making it difficult to force out a last attempt at a rebuttal.

'Before that night and ever since, I only ever wore jeans and trainers to clubs. The night I looked like a slut, I got treated like one—'

I trailed off, my voice barely audible through my sobs. 'At least that's what he told me.'

We sat silently as the weight of my terrible closing statement choked the air out of the room. Could it be true that these 'facts' I'd applied to myself were the voices of others? The messages I had received, consumed and taken as truths during my most vulnerable moments? Paddy had a point about my degrees – I'd seen first-hand how common a practice it was to present data in a favourable way, to massage results to produce a statistically significant outcome. In that moment, I knew but didn't want to admit that perhaps I'd massaged my own data and assigned blame to the wrong places.

Over the two years we worked together, Paddy regularly challenged me on rape myths and my 'logic', before moving on to explore why I believed it to be fact and identifying where my internalised misogyny stemmed from.

To put this in context, below is a list of the comments and responses I have received after disclosing my rapes. Time and time again, I reached out – to male and female friends, family, counsellors and medical professionals – yearning for someone to provide me with the response I needed.

But instead, I placed every negative word, every damaging turn of phrase and every inadequate reaction upon my shoulders, carrying the weight of other people's blame and shame until their voices echoed louder than my own.

1. 'Did you say no?'
2. 'Are you sure you said no?'

3. 'What were you wearing?'
4. 'Had you been drinking?'
5. 'How much had you drunk?'
6. 'Why were you on your own?'
7. 'How could he have sex with you, unless you were turned on?'
8. 'What underwear were you wearing?'
9. 'Why didn't you just keep your knees together?'
10. 'If it happened, why didn't you report it?'
11. 'If it happened, why were you kissing a random bloke two nights later?'
12. 'It's your responsibility to stop him from doing it again to someone else.'
13. 'You're selfish for not reporting it.'
14. 'Do not throw your whole life away over just one misunderstanding.'
15. 'Let me fix you [with sex].'
16. 'You're damaged goods.'
17. 'I'm breaking up with you.'
18. 'You disgust me.'
19. 'You have to go to the police. I won't be able to sleep knowing there's a rapist running around town.'
20. 'Why didn't you run away?'
21. 'Why didn't you fight back?'
22. 'Were you flirting with him?'
23. 'So, you kissed him first, and were attracted to him, but didn't want to shag him? That doesn't make sense.'
24. 'Why would someone do that?'

25. 'Are you sure he meant to?'
26. 'Maybe he got carried away?'
27. 'Blokes do that; it's no big deal.'
28. 'Just get over it.'
29. 'I'm sure it was a misunderstanding. It was probably misinterpreted lust.'
30. 'Are you sure it was [whispers] "rape"?'
31. 'You can't just say no halfway through and expect men to be able to stop.'
32. 'You didn't get yourself pregnant, did you?'
33. 'Sometimes we have to accept responsibility for our own mistakes.'
34. 'Do you have trouble saying no in other areas of your life?'
35. 'You always were a bit of a slut/tease.'
36. 'Maybe he couldn't help it.'
37. 'Did you fancy him?'
38. 'Are you sure?'
39. 'Who was it?'
40. 'That's a pretty big accusation.'
41. 'You have to be careful saying that word; you could ruin someone's life.'
42. 'It doesn't sound like rape if he wore a condom.'
43. 'I thought you were cleverer than this.'
44. 'How could you be so stupid?'
45. 'How could you let this happen?'
46. 'Yeah, right, of course you were.'
47. 'Don't be so dramatic.'

48. 'You're lying.'
49. 'You're covering up because you're too ashamed that you had a one-night stand.'
50. 'If that's true, why isn't he in prison and why are you seeing a male therapist? It's weird.'
51. A slap around the face.
52. A sliced forearm.
53. Laughter.
54. 'This isn't the first time someone has lied to me about being raped.'
55. 'You used the exact same words to describe it as someone on TV.'
56. 'You deserve an Oscar for that performance.'
57. 'Do everyone a favour and kill yourself.'
58. 'Why are you telling me?'
59. 'I can't help you.'
60. Silence.

In one night, my whole world changed. My relationship with X and my friends, my trust in others and myself, all shattered. I became lost. Unable to cope with a new and brutal perspective on the world and the people in it, I turned the blame inwards. It was far easier for me, and for the girlfriends I told, to blame me for being drunk and wearing a short skirt than to admit that someone could be capable of such a heinous act. It was also a convenient truth for them. If this was my fault, they weren't in danger.

Even after two years of therapy, I often slipped back to

thoughts of 'if only I'd been sober or wearing more', ignoring certain facts and selecting those that placed the blame on me. Yes, I was raped while wearing a short skirt, drunk and alone. I was also violently raped while wearing pyjamas with cartoon sheep on them in my own flat. Both times by someone I should have been able to trust.

In addition to the responses I received whenever I disclosed that I'd been raped, there was another facet of my experience where I – along with countless others – were blamed and made to feel responsible for our assaults.

* * *

'I spoke to my friend yesterday about everything that has happened,' I said during one session. 'She asked me if I'd ever considered reporting it.'

From our very first session, Paddy knew that I hadn't reported what had happened.

'How do you feel being asked that?' he said.

'Conflicted, I guess.'

'In what way?'

'I feel that there is an expectation—'

'From?'

'From society, I suppose, to report this stuff. But I'm also painfully aware of the statistics on conviction rates. I looked at them the other day and realised that someone is more likely to get convicted for bicycle theft than rape. I think it was 1.6 per cent for bicycle theft and 1.4 per cent for rape.'

'Those are depressing statistics.'

'Yes, it's almost as if my body is worth less than a bicycle.'

We sat in silence before Paddy spoke again. 'Did you consider reporting it at the time?'

'The night it first happened, I was in shock. I was scared and physically hurt. Everyone seemed angry with me that I wouldn't go to the police, but I just wanted to pretend it hadn't happened and go to bed.' As I said this, I began to notice the flicker of compassion for my eighteen-year-old self. 'In the following days, I kept questioning what had happened, if I'd said "no" clearly enough. I worried that I'd be judged on leaving the club alone and for wearing what I had.'

'You felt your own terror and pain. And everyone's anger. And then you anticipated their judgement.'

'Yes. I was too scared to even tell anyone who it was. He was popular, charming, sporty. I was a drunken mess. At least I was on that night. I had no proof that it wasn't consensual. Although, for some reason, I kept the clothes I was wearing that night for over a year. I burnt them in the end.'

'You don't need to prove it wasn't consensual,' he added quietly.

'I was also terrified I'd get into trouble – that I'd be chucked out of university. People kept trying to make me name him, but I couldn't. Or wouldn't.'

I felt rage building at the loss of control I'd experienced at the time. Embarrassment then swiftly replaced the anger. 'Sorry, that sounds really cowardly.'

'It sounds entirely human. You were scared. Of him. Of

the repercussions of reporting him, the popular guy. Of losing your place at university.'

'And one thing that I don't really understand – for some reason, I didn't want X to get into trouble. He'd gone from being a good friend – I think even the evening before that first time we'd been to the cinema – into something quite different, and I didn't know how to deal with that. In fact, I'm still confused about whether he's a nice person or not.'

'So, there was an abrupt shift. Like a switch being flicked. And it was hard to reconcile one version of X – the friend with whom you shared so much – with the other one. And a part of you remained convinced you would have been reporting your friend to the police.'

I nodded. 'Exactly. I was scared to get into trouble and also scared of getting him into trouble – like maybe his actions were my fault, I suppose.'

'So many people have made you feel responsible for X's actions, Anna.'

Another memory drifted to the surface. 'After the first time, I'd worked really hard to get my life back on track. I managed to get a 2:1 in my first-year exams, despite everything that was going on. But after the second, erm, time – just before I went home for the summer holidays – it completely threw me.'

'That sounds like quite the understatement.'

'Yeah. Anyway, I was physically quite unwell. I kept getting migraines and throwing up.'

'Sounds like your body was reacting to the trauma.'

'Probably. I went to see a doctor. I ended up blurting it out.'

'You told them you'd been raped?'

'Yes, but I didn't mean to. I just didn't know what to do. I knew I couldn't tell any friends – I'd spent months making new ones. Ones that didn't know about the first time. I went to see a doctor on the spur of the moment. I cried and everything. It was humiliating.'

'What was the outcome?'

'Nothing. They gave me some leaflets and helpline numbers. I'm not sure what else they could've done though. A while later, I went to another GP back home as I needed a repeat prescription, but I was ambushed by a discussion about rape and how it was my duty to stop X from hurting anyone else.'

'That feels like a violation. You'd wanted to discuss one thing and suddenly your past was brought up and you were made to feel that, somehow, you are responsible for him.'

'Yes, I was mortified that they knew but also quite cross that it was somehow my responsibility. I was barely keeping myself together – physically – I didn't have the capacity to think about X.'

'You were doing what you needed to do to survive.'

'I suppose deep down I knew what X was and what he had inflicted upon me, but to admit that to anyone was too great a risk. Almost like if I said it aloud, I'd somehow make it happen again? So, I decided to concentrate on myself. Bury it all. Ignore it.'

'That sounds completely understandable, Anna. A necessary but delicate balance to protect yourself.'

CHAPTER 26

'At one time or another, we all try to silence painful emotions. But when we succeed in feeling nothing we lose the only means we have of knowing what hurts us, and why.'
STEPHEN GROSZ, THE EXAMINED LIFE:
HOW WE LOSE AND FIND OURSELVES

ANNA

I try really hard not to lie. With the exception of the magical untruths I tell my children, I'd like to think I am pretty truthful and honest. But, in fact, I lied to myself all the time. I lied to myself for twenty years.

X had always dominated the majority of my therapy sessions and, indeed, he filled my head between appointments and haunted my dreams.

Once the account was written, I became overwhelmed. Triggered and traumatised. So much so that I didn't want to believe my words and the apparent truth of the situation. I began to convince myself that the assaults hadn't happened at all. And if that was the case, then I must be the evil one and he must, of course, be a nice guy.

One night I woke up gasping for air, bolting upright and panicking in the dark. Sam woke too and put a hand on my arm. 'Follow my breathing,' he instructed. I placed my head on his chest and began to focus my attention on the slow movement of his torso. Eventually, my choppy breaths began to fall in sync with his, in a perfect harmony and unspoken understanding.

'Better?' he asked.

'Better,' I said, a little embarrassed. I'd always been taught to hide my pain or minimise it for the comfort of others and allowing people to help me was still an uncomfortable experience.

I glanced at the clock on the bedside table. The red glow showed 2.22 a.m.

'I'm going to check on the kids,' I whispered, although Sam had already fallen back to sleep. Thankful that I hadn't ruined his rest for the night, and not wanting to disturb him further, I tiptoed along the landing, pausing at each child's bedroom door to hear their delicate breaths, and crept downstairs knowing that I wouldn't be able to return to sleep. Part of me was too frightened to do so.

I filled a glass with water, tilting its edge against the cool stream from the tap, trying to be as quiet as possible, and took up my usual nocturnal spot at the kitchen table. I hadn't remembered having a nightmare, but I felt exhausted after the panic attack. *Am I broken? Why can't I let this go?* I paced around the kitchen, feeling a sudden urge to move. *Pull yourself together. You're not broken, you're just a bit damaged. No, not damaged – I hate that word. Maybe I'm just not perfect.* I sat back down at the table and traced the knots on its surface with my index finger. *Even wood has imperfections. Oh, for fuck's sake, stop being a victim. It can't have been that bad. Perhaps I've overreacted? Why would he have hurt me? I must have been mistaken.*

Then an idea popped into my head... *I wonder what he's up to? I wonder where he lives, what his job is, if he has a family?*

I picked up my phone. *Think about this. If I look him up and can see his face without crumbling, then surely that means it wasn't that bad? But if it was that bad, I don't want him to know I've looked him up and I can't risk him finding me.* While I knew that 2.30 a.m. wasn't the best time to launch my investigation, and the quartz-like clarity I'd felt only moments before now felt more like a milky moonstone, I was absolutely compelled. After creating a fake account on a social media app, I carefully typed his name into the search bar. I scrolled through the results I was given: a musician with the same name, a rugby player, a guy in Ohio, several profiles without a photo, and then I stopped as I spotted his face smiling back at me. For a moment, everything seemed to freeze, the already-quiet house descended into a deafening silence. I stopped breathing, stopped thinking. A small whimper involuntarily left my lips as I felt the blood drain from me. I hadn't seen his face for years and now a tsunami of emotions came flooding back. Scared and confused, I closed the app and made my way back upstairs to the security of my bed, chastising myself for being so stupid.

Over the following days, I couldn't stop thinking about the face I'd seen on the profile. I found myself pondering the events I'd painstakingly written about in my account less and less and thinking more about who X might be now. My relentless curiosity pushed me to look again. The next time, as I sat at the kitchen table bathed in the light of a waning moon, I made it onto his profile. I spent the early hours of the morning looking through his photos, being careful not to 'like' any, and constructing an entire fantasy about who he was. From his online persona, he came across as funny, popular, charming. A nice family guy who was married with children. The more I looked at this side of him, the easier it became to block out the side he'd shown me.

Finally, I went back to bed where I succumbed to guilt and confusion and drifted off into a disturbed sleep. Earlier, I'd seen a photo on social media of X on a golf course. Now I dreamt about him driving us both around in a scarlet-red golf buggy. We were smiling and laughing. Happy. He was driving too fast and it was exhilarating. I felt carefree, but the feeling was tinged with a sense of danger. Then, he hit a bump in the grass and the buggy lurched violently to one side. I was thrown from the golf cart and landed, hurt. X didn't stop to help and, instead, drove away, laughing. In my dream, I felt confused, lost and hurt and had woken up even more disorientated at 4 a.m., sweating and groggy, knowing that this was one dream I wouldn't be able to tell Paddy about.

Over the next few weeks, I regularly looked at his profile and managed to find him on other social media platforms. As I scrolled through his posts, I could see that he was charming, witty, self-deprecating, seemingly a perfect gentleman. Everyone seemed to love him and be drawn to him. I could see it in the comments, mostly from young women.

I began to obsessively look up definitions of rape and whether it was possible to have hallucinations. If you search for something long enough, you can usually find what you're looking for. And, indeed, I found multiple explanations for why nothing had in fact happened to me or why, if something had happened, then he couldn't have meant it. I was the one who was mistaken; I didn't make it clear that I hadn't consented. X was the perfect friend and now the perfect family man.

I confidently walked into my next therapy session and sat on the couch, giving Lola a welcome scratch behind her ear.

'I need to apologise,' I began, still stroking Lola and avoiding Paddy's eye. 'I've been looking up definitions of rape and thankfully it doesn't apply to me. Sorry for wasting your time.' I was completely convinced by my statement and I didn't want my therapist to dissuade me.

An awkward silence fell between us. Eventually, the tension reached an unbearable pitch and I slowly raised my head to look at him. Confusion was etched across his face.

PADDY

By now, I was used to the rhythm of our sessions. We'd make headway with Anna's understanding of blame and responsibility, that X was culpable, before Anna would slip back into self-blame, a place that, while painful, was familiar. She had intimated many times that it was far easier for her to blame herself than truly consider the alternative, but she had made progress.

So, I had not anticipated this. Shock rippled through me. It was as if, at a stroke, everything we'd achieved by this point had been wiped away.

'Anna,' I said, the word inadvertently escaping my mouth as a sigh. 'Where has this come from?'

'I don't need to talk about it,' she said abruptly. 'I just wanted to let you know. I'm sorry.'

Silence descended on the room once again. It was weighted with a mixture of disappointment and frustration. Certainly mine and perhaps hers too.

This was completely new territory for me and I was wholly unprepared.

I was used to denial – to clients resisting or refusing to acknowledge the painful reality of their experience. It's a perfectly natural response that helps to protect them from what can feel like unbearable discomfort. Denial is both a shield – to push away dark forces – and a comfort blanket, wrapping them up in a soft but false sense of security. Anna was no stranger to it. She'd existed in that state for decades before seeking therapy. That phase was understandable. But this was something else.

'I'm not angry, Anna.' This felt like an important point to make, as I had probably not managed to hide the note of frustration in my voice. 'But I am genuinely concerned and bewildered.'

'Sam is too,' she said with a slight shrug, as if we were both at fault for failing to see what was obvious to her.

'He keeps asking questions, but I don't know how to answer them.'

There was a rigid stubbornness to her, but at the same time she wriggled uncomfortably on the sofa, as if turmoil was coiled inside her, like a snake.

'Can I ask what the definitions say?' I said eventually, keeping my voice measured, void of the disappointment I felt.

———————— " " ————————

ANNA

Even though I'd written a long Word document compiling all the proof I needed, I didn't want to show Paddy.

'It doesn't matter. I wasn't clear enough. X wasn't a mind reader. Yes, we had sex, but I suppose he just didn't recognise my discomfort.' I carried on quickly before my embarrassment at saying the word 'sex' aloud could register and before Paddy was able to argue. 'I don't know why I've let it affect me so much and for so long. I feel stupid. I can't believe I've accused someone of something so horrible. But now I know that it didn't happen, I can sleep better and dream better.'

———————————— " " ————————————

PADDY

I paused. It felt like she was in such a delicate place. So desperate to hold on to this softer narrative, so scared of the truth. I knew I had to be gentle but also that I had to bring her back to where she'd fought so hard to be.

'Anna,' I said softly, 'did you consent to having sex?'

'I don't think I said "no".'

'You do not have to explicitly spell out "no" for it to be obvious that consent has not been given. And even if X had somehow massively failed to pick up on that message, did you consent to him putting his hand over your mouth or his arm across your throat?'

She visibly shuddered and I hated that I'd induced this reaction. But at the same time, I could not sit by as she threw away all her hard work, the result of her extraordinary courage and fortitude.

'It was rape,' I added. 'On both occasions.'

At my mentioning the second assault, she looked at me and frowned.

'I think the second time must have been a hallucination,' she said, maintaining eye contact, as if daring me to disagree.

Her explanation for the second rape carried with it an air

of desperation. I felt torn inside: aware of the need for truth but aware too that this new narrative had Anna clinging on to a ledge by her fingers. By reminding her of the truth, it felt as if I was peeling those fingers away, sending her hurtling into the abyss.

'Anna, I'm going to word this as gently as I possibly can. Your account of the second rape, which I've read many times now, does not have the quality of a hallucination. It is far too detailed and consistently recalled.'

'OK,' she said, neither agreeing nor disagreeing with me.

---- " " ----

ANNA

His voice seemed so far away and, in my head, I was already in my car leaving the session. Driving away, carefree.

'I don't know what you want me to say.' *I want to leave, but I also can't feel my feet.*

'Your mind may wish to tell you that none of this is true,' he said. 'But your body cannot lie. I've witnessed the blood draining from your face as you've had flashbacks, here in this room. I've guided you through panic attacks at the mere mention of the word "rape", sat with you as you've dissociated when recounting your very long list of physical injuries. Even now, you're wriggling with discomfort.'

Paddy's uncomfortable words floated in the air, bringing me back to reality, back to the room and back to my body.

I sunk into the couch, the fight leaving me. I felt deflated. I could taste blood in my mouth as I realised I'd chewed my lip a little too hard.

'Maybe they were false memories? I've read a lot about them,' I offered, weakly.

'And if they are, who would have put them there, Anna?'

I didn't know the answers and I was irritated that Paddy was challenging me. I'd spent hours and hours researching this and had reached my own conclusions.

———————— " " ————————

PADDY

As the session drew to a close, I made one final comment. She might have her new narrative, but this was a therapeutic relationship. There were two of us in the room, two of us who had been on this journey.

'Anna,' I said. 'I cannot unknow what I know.'

CHAPTER 27

ANNA

In the sessions that followed, I started to pull away from therapy and from Paddy. I'd shut down and become mute. I'd leave early or not say goodbye. He angered me because somewhere deep down, I knew he was right. He was trying to pull me back to my reality. And I wanted to be anywhere but there.

My denial ran so deep that I started to sleep well. I wasn't having panic attacks or flashbacks, and I wasn't self-harming. All of this made me think I was cured.

For several weeks, Paddy consistently tried to help me see X the way he did, but I became more and more resistant. I was reminded of the dream I'd once had about a train, with Paddy at one end and my family at the other. But now, I'd unhooked my therapist's carriage, our beliefs diverging like trains on different tracks. Yet, for some reason, I returned to therapy every week. I could never bring myself to say I'd lied about being raped, because deep down I knew that what had happened was real. So, I'd say to Paddy that perhaps I was mistaken. I couldn't deny that the rapes had occurred, but I could mitigate them so that they weren't horrific incidents that played over and over in my mind.

'I feel like such an evil person for misunderstanding what happened to me – and I know what you'll say to that.'

He smiled. 'I'm curious, what would I say?'

'That I'm not the evil one, X is.'

'OK,' he said, 'but you clearly don't believe that.'

'I believe that *you* think he's evil. But I know for a fact that he isn't.'

'How?'

Shit. Am I going to tell him?

I searched his face, trying to evaluate whether I should, and if I could, tell him. 'I've been looking him up on social media. I have been for a long time.' I fidgeted before adding, 'Sorry.'

'And what did you glean from your research?'

He's not angry that I've been keeping this from him.

Suddenly, my eyes began to well and I could feel the resistance of the past few weeks melting away.

'That he's really happy and charming and nice and *everything*,' I said, through a waterfall of tears.

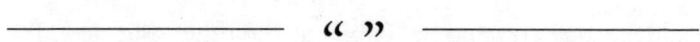

PADDY

At that precise moment, her denial made a little more sense.

She'd found a version of X that was softer than the monster in her dreams. A smiling avatar on social media.

'You see the version of him that he wants to portray to the world, Anna.'

She looked at me with shiny, bloodshot eyes. 'But he's got a wife and kids. He's a nice bloke.'

'There may be some nice aspects to him,' I said. 'No one is solely defined by their worst actions.'

'I don't know any more. I don't know who he is, I don't know who I am. I both know and don't know what happened. I'm so tired of fighting and feeling confused. I'm fed up with navel-gazing. I don't know whether to somehow romanticise it, but then that makes me feel sick. I just want it to never have happened,' she burst out.

At this point, I understood that there was only one way to work. I had the truth in my head, but here, in the room, I had to hold both versions of it for Anna.

Time and again, she returned to the 'facts' she'd gleaned online. The affable-looking guy with his wife, family and friends. The man she remembered from university, a friend with whom she had hung out and watched films, confided in.

'He may be those things,' I'd say at least once every session. 'But he also raped you.'

Every time I did this, I'd watch her face crease with confusion and discomfort.

* * *

One morning, she brought a dream to the session. She was with a child, a little girl who did not belong to her but for whom she cared deeply. The two of them were walking through a city. An alarm went off and everyone apart from Anna and the child began to panic and run into buildings for cover. Eventually, they found themselves on a staircase looking out of a big window at the cityscape below. The streets were a scene of carnage as a monster tore through the crowds, attacking and killing people. Observing the scene, Anna refused to acknowledge what was unravelling in front of her.

'What do you think is happening here?' I asked.

Anna, by now an accomplished dream analyst, thought for a moment.

'The child and I are past and present intermingled,' she said. 'And my present self is refusing to recognise the threat.'

'What does that tell you?'

She looked annoyed, like I'd somehow trapped her. 'I'm in denial.'

There had been many moments of doubt but, until now, nothing as unequivocal as this. She'd finally admitted where she was. But it was a temporary moment of clarity. In the weeks to come, Anna seemed to double down, sinking deeper into denial.

CHAPTER 28

ANNA

Around eighteen months into my therapy journey, I was entrenched in denial and completely convinced that the first incident with X was a misunderstanding and the second was a false memory/dream/hallucination/some other explanation. I was sleeping well and the nightmares, flashbacks and panic attacks had stopped. I'd persuaded myself that it hadn't happened and therefore I couldn't be traumatised. I was also certain that if I visited my old university city, I could prove to myself that these memories were indeed false. I didn't have an explanation for why I had false memories but believed that being in Bristol might help me establish that.

I suggested this to Paddy one session. 'I've been thinking about visiting Bristol,' I said, nervously. While I'd been considering the idea for weeks, it was news to him.

He took a deep breath, uncrossed his legs and carefully selected his next words. 'I have to tell you that I have concerns.'

Although his voice remained calm and measured, his body

language open and diplomatic, I knew him well enough to notice his subtle signs of discomfort. His hand reached up to rub his neck and a grimace flickered across his face.

'What would you hope to achieve by going back there?' he asked.

'I just have to find out if those flashbacks were real. If I visit Bristol, I think I can figure it all out and prove to myself that nothing happened.'

'Anna,' he said, 'I know that we have two different perspectives on the events and I want to make sure that I stay within your frame of reference. But also I wouldn't be congruent if I didn't tell you I'm worried about what you're contemplating.'

'You don't need to be worried, nothing happened to me,' I said swiftly, irritation inflecting my still-polite reply.

He held up his palms. 'OK, I hear what you're saying, but just for a moment let's look at this in a different way. If there is even a slight chance that these events did happen, I'm worried that you could be retraumatised in the middle of a city. And also that you'd be alone.'

'I don't want anyone with me,' I said abruptly.

'Because...?'

'Because I don't want an audience if I do get traumatised or have a panic attack. I don't want to have to think about anyone else's emotions. I couldn't take Sam or a friend, even though they've already offered, because I'd be too worried about them. I also don't want the pressure of going all the way there and then feeling like I have to go through with it.'

'In case you change your mind?'

'Exactly. I think I know what I'd do and where I'd go, but if I freak out and panic, I'd feel pressured into doing it anyway, just to please others.'

We sat in a muted atmosphere for a few minutes before Paddy spoke.

'What about me? I'm not sure how it would work, but maybe we could meet there?'

Oh God, no. 'Thank you, but no. Really, really, no,' I replied, adamantly.

———————— " " ————————

PADDY

The first time Anna raised the idea of visiting Bristol, I was, frankly, horrified. She'd been retraumatised many times in sessions, reliving the horror of her ordeals within the safety of the counselling room. Panic would cloud her face, she'd pale and I could only imagine the speed at which her heart was racing. But in that safe space, I could ease Anna gently back into the here and now by asking her to anchor herself on an object in the room, the sound of my voice or the birdsong outside, and bring her pulse under control by encouraging her to breathe until she calmed.

In Bristol on her own, there was no safety net to fall into. She was in such a state of deep denial, the truth would hit her like a freight train. I pictured her in the street, staring up at an innocuous building while inside her own foundations crumbled and, brick by brick, she collapsed onto the pavement.

I could not let this happen.

---- " " ----

ANNA

As I left the session and walked down the country lane, Paddy's offer echoed in my head. I climbed inside my car and shut the door. Peace. Usually, I drove away immediately, keen to get home to Sam and the kids, but that day I closed my eyes and sat thinking about my potential trip. While I appreciated Paddy's offer, I needed to do this alone. What happened was a misunderstanding and a false memory. I didn't want anyone questioning me. I knew Paddy and I had different views and I didn't want any other opinions in my head. I also didn't need him to tell me that X wasn't the nice guy I believed him to be.

* * *

That night I dreamt. Acres of land had been slashed and burnt for farming. I saw myself walking through the ashes and weaving through the remains of trees that had been cruelly hacked. I ran to the top of a hill where I found one remaining tree. It was a large oak with strong roots. A swing hung from one of the branches and I sat down. As I started to swing, I felt calm, but I also knew I was blocking out the destruction and the fires that were creeping up behind me. The ground beneath my feet was crumbling and falling into what appeared to be the endless darkness below. And then I spotted another hill across from me. Paddy was there, standing next to a long line of people. I sensed I knew them all, but I couldn't see their faces.

'Just swing across and jump,' Paddy said.

But I smiled and shook my head. I had no intention of crossing the chasm. What if I fell?

CHAPTER 29

PADDY

Not long after Anna first mentioned travelling to Bristol by herself, Covid-19 swept through the nation and, in March 2020, we were forced into lockdown. For the foreseeable future, Anna wasn't going anywhere except around her village.

Unwelcome and unsettling though the pandemic was, it was a huge relief to know that she was grounded and couldn't just leap in her car and speed up the M5 to a very uncertain encounter with her past. Ultimately, lockdown was a gift which allowed us to consider a trip in a more measured way. A way that ultimately gave her the resolution she truly needed.

———————— " " ————————

ANNA

As the likelihood of a trip was put on hold, Paddy and I had a chance to discuss the *potential* of a trip. How would it work?

What was I hoping to achieve? During these conversations, Paddy repeated his offer to accompany me, which I continued to decline.

'I'm wondering if there's another reason why you don't want me with you in Bristol?' he said during one session. 'Perhaps there's a fear I might contradict the view that you're currently holding on to about X?'

I chewed my lip, while a sinking feeling in my stomach indicated that he was correct.

'Maybe.' *Definitely*.

'So, let me ask you a question, Anna. If you're so convinced that the events didn't happen and that X isn't a rapist, then what's the point in going to Bristol?'

Fuck, he has a point.

I couldn't answer, but it was a thought that stayed in my head.

And then, something happened that I did not expect.

Although I was sleeping well and not self-harming, flashbacks had begun to creep back into my seemingly happy life.

Just before lockdown, I went out for dinner with Sam, without the children, which was a rarity. Towards the end of the night, I went to find the loo and as soon as I opened the door, I was greeted by a specific design of tiles on the floor. Immediately, a surge of electricity pulsed through my veins and my vision tunnelled into pinpoint focus. Vomit clawed its way up my throat. I stumbled back to the table, managing to push the panic aside and continue the evening, but I was confused. I was certain that the rapes hadn't happened, so why was I so viscerally affected by the tiles? The same tiles that had been on the floor of the bathroom in my student flat.

On another occasion, I froze in terror at the sight of a rack of belts in a shop before running out in embarrassment. I became unable to wear necklaces or scarves for fear of choking, as memories of X's arm over my throat forced their way into my brain in ultra-high definition.

Why were these everyday objects having such an effect on me? It felt like something was building and waiting to emerge. And when it did, it changed everything.

The confusing images and reactions had been growing for months. Sometimes, I'd share them with Paddy, but I was mostly alone in my confusion and pain. I had disconnected from therapy and from my therapist.

Then, one Sunday morning, I woke with my head pounding, vision blurred, and made my way to the toilet where I was violently sick. My memory of the next twelve to fourteen hours is hazy, but I effectively became trapped inside continuous flashbacks, reliving every moment of the events from twenty years ago. Sam checked on me throughout the day. He believed that I had a migraine but was concerned. Unable to communicate what was going on, I was ultimately alone. He'd taken the children to a family party for several hours. Later, he told me he had arrived home to find me on the bathroom floor, cold, shivering and covered in sweat.

Minutes felt like an eternity and yet the hours flew by. Eventually I emerged, confused at how daylight was now darkness. I made my way downstairs and ate before returning to bed and sleeping heavily with my head on Sam's chest until the alarm rang the next day.

Scared but also feeling very ill, I cancelled my appointment with Paddy for the first time. After the wonderful chaos and distraction of the school runs, I sat at home, alone, with the shutters closed, terrified of my new reality. I had remembered *everything*. Every detail, every physical pain and every emotion that had accompanied it. I could no longer deny that the rapes had happened. I felt battered, completely adrift. Lost.

Paddy emailed to ask if I wanted to rearrange and out of politeness, obligation or sheer desperation, I agreed to return.

A few days later, I sat in front of him. I was broken. My previous certainties shattered by truth. Unable to deny what X was and what he had inflicted upon me, I didn't want to argue with Paddy and I was finally ready to receive the compassion I'd resisted for months.

I briefly explained to him what had happened on that Sunday. Well, as much as I could remember, and how it had left me with a stark new reality. All fight had been cruelly taken from me. It was like I was eighteen again, had been through the infernos of hell and was now sitting, burnt and smoking, on Paddy's couch.

———————————— " " ————————————

PADDY

I didn't want Anna to be back where she'd started: barely

sleeping, in the grip of terrifying flashbacks and triggered by objects that reduced her to a shaking, sweating shell of a woman.

At the same time, I was relieved. Yes, she was feeling all the cruel and debilitating symptoms that had first brought her to therapy, but I was also convinced that this was progress. It was as if her unconscious had taken a sledgehammer to the narrative of denial she'd so carefully constructed.

'I'm so sorry that you had to endure that, Anna,' I said.

'Yeah. Guess I'm out of denial then.'

'Yes, but for it to have happened in that way. It sounds terrifying.'

'Yeah,' she shrugged. 'X isn't a nice person.'

'No, he's not.'

I looked at Anna, assessing her state. She appeared crushed and tired but not defeated. I sensed a rare opportunity, where it might just be possible to get her to not only embrace the truth of what had happened but say it out loud in a way that would prove to be lastingly powerful. The conversation that follows might sound cruel, but I was convinced that Anna needed to hear herself.

———————— " " ————————

ANNA

'What did X do to you, Anna?'

'He... hurt me.'

'Yes, he did. *How* did he hurt you, Anna?'

'He—' I began, but I couldn't finish the sentence. I tried again, 'He... I think... he... Oh, for fuck's sake, I can't say it,' I said, the frustration impeding me.

'I know that this is incredibly hard for you, Anna. But I think that if you can finally acknowledge what he is and what he did to you, if you can say just three words, it could be a huge step.'

'But if I say it, I can't *unsay* it.'

I looked across the room to the map on the wall, my safe place when things got too hard. I took a deep breath and met Paddy's eyes in a silent exchange. There were so many times I wished I could rewrite the past and one of my deepest regrets was telling a friend after the first rape. I'd replayed my exchange with them incessantly, wishing I could take back the words that set off a chain of events. Uttering them now would make it real. I wouldn't be able to hide behind the veil of denial and I'd have to face everything that terrified me. The word I'd evaded all these years had caused harm, division and destruction. But perhaps it could also do the opposite?

A sense of timelessness descended, as though there was only this moment and the two of us. The air in the room almost crackled with anticipation. I knew what I needed to do. To say. I knew Paddy was rooting for me.

'He raped me.'

My head immediately dipped, but pure willpower forced me to lift it and meet Paddy's gaze. I refused to go backwards now.

'Yes, he did.'

PADDY

It had taken a year and a half to get here. During that time, we had collectively uttered thousands of words: in the phone messages Anna asked me to read when terror and shame had stolen her voice; in the emails, where she found a way to explore or clarify the thoughts that she could not access in the room with me; and in the sessions, as her strength and confidence gradually grew.

But in all that time, no words were expressed with quite the power of the three she uttered that day.

Anna had been clinging on to a ledge; her body dangling over an abyss. Of course she didn't want to relinquish her grip – monsters lay below. But in that moment, I think she realised that they were less terrifying than the ones she kept alive by hanging on.

And so, she loosened her fingers and let herself drop, knowing, I hope, that I was with her.

CHAPTER 30

ANNA

About four months after I'd first suggested the trip, we returned to the discussion. Lockdown had returned me to my pre-denial state.

'Hypothetically, if I accepted your offer to come with me on the trip, erm, how would it work?'

'*Hypothetically*,' he said, smiling, 'I suggest that we travel separately and meet there.'

'I don't think I want to be alone in Bristol. I'm tired of pretending I can do everything by myself.'

'My offer stands, Anna.'

———————————— " " ————————————

PADDY

That period of time, when the nation ground to a halt, was productive for us. But I don't think Anna necessarily saw it that way at the time. The story she'd led herself to believe out of a desperate desire not to see or feel the truth was gone and a painful process of facing it, and what it meant, began again. This was accompanied by the pendulum swing she'd always experienced as she lurched between blaming herself and her perpetrator, and between her need for self-care and her desire to self-harm.

It was like we had to go backwards to go forwards.

So, when she returned to the idea of the trip, although it was unknown territory, it felt like a moment of hope.

———————————— " " ————————————

ANNA

I returned the next week prepared.

'If the offer still stands, I'd appreciate you meeting me in Bristol,' I started, keen to get it out of the way.

'Of course.'

I leant over and handed Paddy a plastic wallet full of printouts.

'In that case,' I said, 'I've been researching—'

Paddy smiled wryly. He was familiar with my way of working by now.

'And I found a couple of journal articles from therapists who have attempted similar trips with their clients. From what I can see, they're mostly CBT-based, but I don't see why we can't apply some of the same logic.'

'They sound very interesting. And how was it to look into this?'

I smiled. He understood. There was comfort, even joy, for me in planning. In finding a degree of control again.

'It was actually OK. I might have even enjoyed it.'

'I spoke to Sue about this last week,' he said.

This was a surprise. I was unsure how invested he was in the idea.

'We talked about taking this room with us to Bristol, so that whatever you discover there can be held within the safe space we've created here.'

'Makes perfect sense,' I nodded.

---------- " " ----------

PADDY

From the moment she began counselling, Anna had held the few things that were in her control in a vice-like grip: the details she was willing to share; the words she was prepared to use; the words she allowed me to use. With her alternative version of the truth shattered, she had been forced to live with all the chaos and pain that this veracity had brought, and her one comfort was the certainty I was close by.

Now she was considering the trip, Anna appeared enthused, an unmistakable confidence and energy in the way she spoke. So long a prisoner of her past, her horrific ordeals robbing her of her voice, sleep and hope, she was in control again. And it made her feel good.

To get us used to a 'mobile' counselling room that we could take to Bristol, I suggested walking sessions. Therapy conducted outdoors had become hugely popular during lockdown. In various professional journals, therapists acknowledged the potential pitfalls – capricious weather, encountering other people who might want to interact, prompting awkward conversations and bursting the bubble – but wrote enthusiastically of the benefits. Clients experienced the boundless sky above their heads – that sense of perspective and possibility – the cycle of nature around them, which brought with it an awareness that decay is always followed by rebirth, and the opportunity to enjoy the soothing sights and sounds of the countryside.

For Anna and me, being outdoors was not about the healing power of nature. Our ultimate destination was a city centre, so the aim of walking was simply to get us used to being in motion.

I remember our first experiment. In the counselling room, Lola had been a near-constant presence, the gentlest of Labradors who, in her soft, serene way, offered Anna a canine version of acceptance and unconditional positive regard. Now, she joined us on the lead. As she calmly led, Anna and I followed, silent at first, while we got accustomed to the feeling of movement together.

I was soon breathless, not so much from the steep climb

but from nerves. It felt unsettling to be outside. The counselling room was my safe space too, somewhere that defined me as a professional, that gave my practice a solid, familiar and physically boundaried context. Outside, I felt untethered, powerless without the walls around me and the prop of my old leather armchair.

But this in itself was a useful experience. In Bristol, I would be similarly exposed, so I needed to get used to the change in environment, the sense of a world unfurling around us, rather than the static backdrop of my room.

That first stroll lasted around twenty minutes, but as we gained confidence, the walks lengthened. Even when we trekked in silence, it still felt helpful. We were growing used to the idea of preserving a therapeutic space while moving outdoors.

But the Devon countryside is a quiet place, so at the back of my mind I couldn't help worrying what it would be like to try to replicate that delicate bubble in a noisy, bustling city centre.

———————— " " ————————

ANNA

As we left the familiarity of the counselling room, Lola trotting ahead of us, I felt calm – relaxed, even. It was a subtle and very welcome departure from the intensity of directly facing each other, to a more casual and companionable situation. We walked in silence for a while, taking in the first signs of spring – the crocuses and snowdrops beginning to emerge, the pleasing return of sunshine – before we briefly chatted about my interest in photographing the landscape. The nature of our conversation didn't seem important, but the exercise itself had proved useful. By now, we could switch between having a casual conversation and being in a more professional setting with ease. If we were going to attempt the trip to Bristol, this was a skill that would serve us well.

The walk gave us both a much-needed confidence boost. And as the weeks passed, I planned for every eventuality. I made spreadsheets consisting of the trip's aims and potential risks. I wanted to ensure that I was as ready as I could be, but I also wanted Paddy to feel as equipped as possible; I knew this was a risk for him too.

Here are the spreadsheets I prepared. Looking back now, I see my need to control the unknown. Within the confines of the rigid rows and columns, there is the reassurance I so desperately needed.

What I am bringing	What I need you to bring
I will be nervous. Terrified, even. But this is something that I really feel the need to do. I'll also be bringing my usual baggage: - Blame - Self-doubt - Shame - Guilt - Humiliation - Fear - Sadness - Self-hate - Anger - Trauma - Regret - Grief and loss - Pain - Anxiety - Self-disappointment - Hurt - Crying - Denial - Disbelief - Despair - No hope - No control - Probable withdrawal - Vulnerability - Hopefully, courage and tenacity	I need you to be challenging and to also recognise when I'm reaching my threshold. Keep me talking and keep talking to me. - Safety - Trust - Core conditions - Compassion - Honesty, congruence and transparency - Encouragement and help to confront feelings/emotions - Motivation - Facilitation - Insight - Help me grow - Validation – of events as well as emotions. If you believe me, tell me - Perspective - Space and patience to work things out for myself - Help me to stay in the present as much as possible - Calm and interventions with panic attacks and dissociation - Courage - Belief - Hope and yet be realistic - Positivity - Achievement - Humour and lighter moments

Fears		How to alleviate
Rational	That I'll become overwhelmed – panic and/or dissociate: • Embarrassment • Guilt • Wasted trip if I dissociate	Follow plans in the tables below. I am reassured that if I panic, you can help calm me down. Help to identify when I am dissociating. Take photos, write notes to help if I have memory lapses.
	Crying.	You have seen me cry now. I feel OK about this.
	I'll withdraw and not communicate verbally.	Keep talking to me. Tell me if you think I'm dissociating.
	I'm scared to be vulnerable.	I'm not expecting anything of you, but I need to pin this fear down.
	Scared to be not in control but think it may be necessary?	Ditto.
	Scared that I may become angry?	Ditto.
	Time pressures if I have a panic attack.	Ditto.
	Fears over new memories or details appearing.	I'm willing to take the risk.
	That the trip will send me into a depressive state/trauma symptoms are exacerbated.	I am aware of this and willing to take the risk. I will try to remain optimistic yet realistic.
	That things will look different from my memories and therefore I will question myself and what happened.	You can tell me that, although the city may have changed in appearance, it doesn't invalidate my experience.

Irrational	That you will leave me if I panic, dissociate, cry or become angry.	I know you won't, but I still need to articulate the fear.
	You will question the validity of my story and think I'm a liar.	Ditto.
	You will blame me.	Ditto.
	You will take X's side.	Ditto.
	You will pity me and think I am weak.	Ditto.

Situation	What might happen	What I can do
Dissociation	Prone to dissociating when overwhelmed. However, I appreciate that some level of dissociation may be necessary when recounting traumatic events. E.g. looking at the events from a safe distance (looking down on myself or X).	Attempt to be aware of signs I'm dissociating – tunnel vision, floaty, people and sounds far away. Unable to move, think or feel. Remember that it will pass.

Helpful actions or interventions by you	Unhelpful interventions
Notice signs of dissociation – you may have to fill in this part – staring into space? Unresponsive? Not listening?	I'm not expecting an unhelpful response.
Help bring me back to the present – ask questions to engage the thinking part of my brain. Ask me to describe surroundings? What can you see? Hear? Although don't ask me too many questions at once.	
Tell me if you think I'm dissociating. Name it. Bring attention to it.	
Connect me to you and to my surroundings.	
Be firm, get my attention. Get me to look at you. Tell me to do something – sit down, stand up, get me to move, drink water?	
Gauge level of dissociation – if you ask me a question and I don't respond, I am possibly dissociating more than if I respond but don't know what the question was. At least I will have recognised that you are there, even if I haven't been listening. Perhaps ask me what is the last thing I remember you asking me?	
Encourage me to explore feelings and delve deeper past phrases such as 'I don't know' or 'I don't feel anything'.	
We need to find a balance between accessing emotions and being overwhelmed by them.	
Ask me to talk about my children, husband or even my dog.	
Please stay with me.	

Situation	What might happen	What I can do
Panic attack	Panic attack, especially during flashbacks/ recounting events. Main symptoms: for me, changes in breathing pattern. Forgetting how to breathe or swallow. Feeling like I'm being strangled. Racing heart, feeling faint. Usually last a few minutes, some have lasted just under fifteen minutes. I haven't had a full panic attack when I have been with you so far, so I'm hoping it is unlikely that I'll have a prolonged attack.	Try to notice surroundings. Breathe out. Know it will pass. Don't push away help. I may be able to bring it under control alone and may not need assistance, but I will need to know you are nearby. Don't try to resist the panic?
Self-harm	I will not engage in self-harming behaviour during the site visit. I have not previously felt the need to utilise this coping strategy when I am with you.	Express verbally painful emotions, as per the past two years. I will be honest and inform you if I am feeling the need to self-harm, so that a discussion can occur.

Helpful actions or interventions by you	Unhelpful interventions
Stay with me. Stay calm. If I am unable to control it by myself, I would like you to use helpful phrases to remind me that you are still there with me, that I'm safe, that it's OK etc. Encourage me to breathe out, perhaps get me to match your breathing. Maybe point out that it's a panic attack. And that while it feels awful, it will pass and I'll be OK. And that you aren't going anywhere. Draw my attention to surroundings – things I can see, hear, touch etc. Reminders that I'm safe with you. That you will stay with me. Reminder that it will pass, that I've survived every one before. Reminders not to resist? Talk to me about my children, husband or even my dog. Help to think of a safe space – like the therapy room?	I honestly don't know, but I feel as though it may possibly be unhelpful to mention X's name – just during a panic attack. E.g. don't say 'He/X isn't here now' or 'He/X can't hurt you.' If I'm having a flashback, he very much feels like he is in the present, so I think it may be confusing. Maybe don't ask me questions because I won't be able to respond?
If I tell you I am having urges but do not want to act upon them: encourage me to talk about the origin of the pain? What the emotion is behind the desire to self-harm in that moment? E.g. anger? At whom? Self-hatred? Punishment? Not wanting to feel emotion? Wanting to feel something? If that doesn't help, distractions? Encouragement of releasing feelings and emotions regularly so that they do not build up.	I'm not expecting an unhelpful response.

PADDY

I'll admit, spreadsheets are not my strong suit, so when Anna took the lead, I felt a degree of relief. However, we discussed every point and every last possible implication of our trip.

Outside of our sessions, I continued to talk through the trip with Sue. With her measured, gently probing manner, she was exactly the sounding board I needed.

Sue described a successful trauma site visit she had made with a client. It was more local, but it had also involved a car journey with the client and occupying new spaces while maintaining the bubble of the counselling room. It was comforting to hear her story. The message I received was that site visits, although not common, were possible and had the potential to bring about change. Increasingly, the trip, while a risk, felt like a calculated one.

We were doing everything possible to adequately prepare, but there were still many moments when I stared at the spreadsheets and felt my stomach twist with anxiety. I was looking at a series of hypothetical situations safely contained within a framework of columns and tables. In Bristol, we would be out in the wild with no protection.

———————————— " " ————————————

ANNA

In the months before the summer of 2020, we were able

to further build up the armour and resources that I knew I would need in Bristol, and shortly before the lockdown restrictions lifted, I spoke to a friend about the trip.

'Wow, I can't believe you're actually going to go back there!' she said, genuinely surprised.

My bravery faltered. Was this a stupid idea? Was I risking retraumatisation?

'You must really trust Paddy,' she continued. And for the very first time, almost two years after our first session, I realised that I did.

When the restrictions were finally rescinded, the public were once again allowed to travel around the UK. As people started making plans to see their loved ones, Paddy and I readied ourselves for departure and a very different kind of trip.

———————————— " " ————————————

PADDY

Although public transport was now available, the possibility of catching Covid was still very real, so we made the decision to travel together. It was not just about minimising the risk of catching an infectious disease and passing it on to my elderly parents; there was also the understanding that travelling alone to Bristol might be traumatic for Anna. And if I was delayed, she might find herself alone in the city.

We decided to break the trip into sections. There was the journey there, during which we agreed to keep our topics of conversation light until we were half an hour from our destination, at which point we would mentally prepare ourselves. Then there was the work we would do in the city itself, and decompression on the way home.

We were as prepared as we could be.

———————————— " " ————————————

ANNA

The night before our trip, I glanced down at the faded patterns on my forearm, my eyes tracing the jagged silvery lines. By now, Paddy had seen the story etched there many times and had not turned away. Each time I had inadvertently revealed the scars, there was a quiet respect and an unspoken acknowledgement of the courage it took to wear my pain so openly.

I hoped, in time, that each scar would represent a moment of courage or resilience in my journey, but for now, all I could see was a constant reminder of pain. And my disgust soon turned to shame.

I looked up the weather forecast for Bristol, hoping for rain or at least a cool temperature. I wanted the excuse to wear clothes that were light and flowy, with each fold keeping my secret. My heart sank as a high of 26°C was predicted for the following day.

We had important work to do. I wanted to be comfortable, but I was spending the best part of the day with Paddy, and if my arms were exposed for the duration, rather than briefly glimpsed as they occasionally were in sessions, I needed to know he'd be comfortable too.

I sent a panicked email to Paddy, covering this concern and a couple of other things that were on my mind.

> Hi Paddy,
>
> I just wanted to check a couple of things before tomorrow:
>
> I think the weather is going to be hot, so I wanted to ask if you'd be OK if I wore short sleeves, which obviously means you'll be able to see my scarred arm. I'm pretty sure I know what your answer will be, but just wanted to check that my scars won't make you uncomfortable.
>
> As I've mentioned before, I'm completely happy for you to tell your family whatever information you need to about the trip and about me.
>
> I'll give you Sam's number, in case of emergency.
>
> I would really like it if the work we have done, and are about to do, could be beneficial to both counsellors and clients. Perhaps you could contact Hannah Murray, the researcher who wrote the paper on trauma visits? I'd be happy for you to do that and to find out whether we can make a useful contribution.
>
> As I'm sure you've seen in the news recently, the number of prosecutions and convictions for rape is at its lowest level since annual recording began. I think that people may have to look at new ways to find resolution and closure. And my best hope is that returning to the scene of trauma, together with therapy, can go some way towards achieving this, for some.

" "

PADDY

Anna was referring to a particular research paper that she'd brought to a session. 'Clients' Experiences of Returning to the Trauma Site during PTSD Treatment: An Exploratory Study', written by psychologists Hannah Murray, Chris Merritt and Nick Grey, looked at the experience of twenty-five people who participated in site visits (as part of trauma-focused CBT for PTSD) and whether they found them helpful. Anna mentioned whether we could contribute to this work by offering our knowledge to the researchers. As it transpired, her motivation formed the foundations of this book. At the time, I took her suggestion as a sign of optimism. She wanted to turn her experience, and what she hoped would be a key element of her recovery, into something that could help others.

This desire struck me as hopeful, because bound up in her proposal was the belief that her recovery was possible.

Her comment about telling my family also seemed positive. Anna no longer felt shame about being in therapy.

That evening, to distract myself from nerves, I drafted an email to Hannah Murray. I laboured over the sentences, struggling to articulate what felt like a perfectly simple offer to support her work.

I couldn't tell if I was tired or simply nervous about the next day. I put my laptop to one side and began to wonder whether it was something else. By contacting the researcher, were we simply heaping an extra layer of pressure on us both? Would we end up (even unconsciously) attempting to shape the visit so that it was useful to the research – and to others who had experienced a similar trauma to Anna – when the only person it needed to benefit at this point was her?

I put this in an email to Anna and she agreed. We decided, at least for now, that we would focus on the trip and what she could get out of it. I also took the opportunity to reassure Anna that, as ever, the sight of her arm would in no way be an issue for me – that my acceptance of her would not change.

Attached to Anna's reply was a finalised document that included where we would park, the places she wanted to visit and a list of aims for the trip and beyond.

———————————— " " ————————————

ANNA

We'd spent months preparing for this expedition. What was I hoping to achieve? What could go wrong? Did the benefits outweigh the risks? This was a collaboration and I trusted and had confidence in my therapist. I also knew that I had certain strengths in the areas of planning and paperwork and realised that if I could take some of this pressure off Paddy, he would be more able to focus on supporting me.

Plans and practicalities:

Park at NCP.

I want to visit the site where the first incident occurred, which is a short walk from the car park. And then trace my steps to my former halls of residence, which are also close by.

I believe that the nightclub I've often mentioned no longer exists, so it may be helpful to recognise that things have changed and moved on and that events are in the past? I wonder if it would be helpful to take photos for future use, but I am undecided whether I'd like you to take them or to take them myself. At this moment, I don't think I'll be able to, but I don't know how I will feel on the day. Or whether there may be some therapeutic benefit in taking them myself?

I'd like, if possible, to walk around the outside of the halls of residence. I am realistic about how much we will be able to access; however, I think I will be able to do some useful work just by being in the vicinity. I've checked Google Street View and I think I will be able to see the halls from the road anyway. There's also a car park at the rear, from which I should be able to see my flat. I cannot remember how to access this car park, but I'm hoping we can figure it out on the day or at least get close to it.

There are a number of large parks very nearby, which may be helpful to retreat to if I become overwhelmed or we wish to talk and decompress, away from the scene.

Aims of the trip:
- Filling in gaps in memories
- Being able to see finer details
- Acknowledging trauma to myself
- Validating trauma and memories to myself
- Acknowledging what X is and what he did
- Being able to say it out loud?
- Achievement of being able to visit a place I have avoided for eighteen years
- Leaving the trauma in the city
- To have the reactions I should have been given from others, from you? Compassion, validation, belief etc.?
- To experience the emotions I should have been allowed to have at the time

Optimistic aims for the future:
- Putting events in the past
- Converting traumatic memories to long-term memories
- Being able to look at events objectively and from a distance
- Not being overwhelmed by events
- Removal of self-blame and shame
- Being able to move on and reclaim my life
- Being able to recognise that X is one person, not the two versions I sometimes hold in my head
- Resolution and closure
- Resulting in a decrease in nightmares, flashbacks, panic attacks, self-harm

PADDY

Here they were, her aims briskly set out as bullet points like an agenda for a meeting.

Some clients begin therapy with a clearly defined goal – to feel happy, to feel less angry, to communicate more effectively with their partner, to process a bereavement. Over the weeks and months that follow, those goals may shift or even become redundant as clients gain a richer understanding of themselves and what they really need.

Anna had been in therapy for almost two years by this point. We'd done the gentle coaxing of her voice, the analysis of her dreams, the painstaking, brick-by-brick building of her account. She knew exactly what she needed.

Anna deserved to achieve every one of the goals she'd set out in the email, to finally feel the loosening of her shackles. I hoped more than anything that the trip delivered results. Results that were every bit as tangible as her goals.

But there were no guarantees and I was only too aware of the trip's potential to disappoint. In the early hours of the morning on the very day we were due to travel, I began to worry about what shape that disappointment might take and how hard it would be, after all her hard work, for Anna to tolerate.

CHAPTER 31

'One day he told me that he'd spent his adulthood trying to let go of his past, and he remarked how ironic it was that he had to get closer to it in order to let it go.'
BESSEL VAN DER KOLK, THE BODY KEEPS THE SCORE: BRAIN, MIND, AND BODY IN THE HEALING OF TRAUMA

Bristol, July 2020

ANNA

As I leave the bar, remembering the route I took twenty years ago, there is a fragile balance between the past, the present and what the future might hold. My courage begins to falter once again and I increase my pace just in case I'm not brave enough to continue on to the next part of our journey. As I retrace my steps from that night, I become more and more anxious. Like a tempest coursing through my body, the adrenaline builds, making my breath quicken and my heart pound with a force I'm sure Paddy can hear. Once again, I'm thankful I'm not alone.

As we make our final turn down a quieter road, we approach the site of my first attack. My steps are suddenly heavy with uncertainty. I begin to slow down. This is the moment I've been dreading. At least at the flats, I had some distance. This place is right in front of me. I can even stand on the spot I was raped, if I want to.

———————————— " " ————————————

PADDY

We've been to the grim-looking halls. The empty bar, the whiff of alcohol hanging in the air and the ghostly trace of raucous students. This is an innocuous-looking green space by a church. It looks like nothing significant, yet when I glance at Anna's face, alabaster white, I know it hums with a malevolent energy.

———————————— " " ————————————

ANNA

I step cautiously into the road and begin to walk across but stop right in the middle. Paralysed. I'm on a precipice about to fall, or about to run headfirst into the final battle. I have no idea whether I'll conquer or fail, but I know that I feel more equipped than ever before, with the totality of our work together acting as my armour. And I'm confident that Paddy is ready to pull me out of the situation if I get into trouble and retreat us to safer ground.

I realise that I'm still standing in the middle of the road.

'Sorry,' I mutter, as a cyclist has to manoeuvre around me.

As we get a little closer, I start to recount what happened on that night. I don't intend to, but I feel an overwhelming need to do so. I'm not even sure who I'm telling it to. As I'm relating the events, people are walking around, keen to reach their own destinations.

———————————— " " ————————————

PADDY

As Anna speaks, I'm suddenly reminded of the couch at the Freud Museum in north London. It's draped with a Persian rug and piled with embroidered cushions. It's where the psychoanalyst's patients would lie – him seated on a chair behind their heads – and, unencumbered by the sight of his physical presence, would unburden themselves in what he hoped was an uncensored stream of unconsciousness.

There's something of that about her delivery now. I've heard the story before, but it sounds different today. The words are flowing out of her, a fast-moving river. They're spoken as the memories surface. It's as if she's purging herself.

ANNA

My brain transforms every man I see in the near vicinity into X, even those who don't look anything like him. Physically, I feel very much in the present, but my mind keeps flashing back to the past, and they are converging. It feels a little like when I suffer from sleep paralysis and I wake up seeing someone standing by my bed. I know that they aren't really there, so I just wait for them to disappear and for me to wake up fully. In this moment, I can see X walking towards me and my body responds accordingly. Rationally, I know it isn't him and I wait for my brain to catch up and realise that too. I can't communicate this to Paddy, but I know he's picking up on my anxiety. I wonder if I've made a mistake coming here, but I'm unwilling to admit defeat just yet.

We walk closer to the spot and I'm suddenly aware of a lot of people. Too many. Some builders nearby are using a pneumatic drill and the chaotic sound pierces my brain and creates a disorientating assault on my senses. My surroundings begin to overwhelm me: people, noises, memories. The air is thick with the residue of pain and I start to panic. Every intake of breath becomes jagged, individual sounds blend together into a distorted and muffled roar. The grass beneath my feet begins to sway and my old companion, nausea, rushes up to greet me.

PADDY

This is exactly the kind of moment we've prepared for, when the life of the city collides with our trip. Outside the bar, the drunken man being tended to by paramedics turned out to be a fleeting moment and was over before we even entered the building. Once inside, we could do what we needed to do reasonably undisturbed. The pneumatic drill is all-pervasive, the least relaxing sound I can imagine at the very moment when Anna needs calm and peace. I'm also aware of the builders' gender. I can't help feeling that their overt masculinity and physicality – the way one of them operates the pneumatic drill almost like it's a weapon – will feel threatening to Anna at this precise moment.

Sure enough, her torrent of words suddenly dries up.

I'm worried that the lid she's pulled from the bunker in her head will soon be slammed shut, sealing in the demons she was so close to expunging.

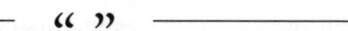

ANNA

'Do you want to move away from the men?' Paddy asks, nodding towards the builders.

I notice that he says 'men' and not 'people'. I've never been fearful of the opposite sex, but in that moment, with the exception of Paddy, I realise that I genuinely am.

I fear that if I open my mouth to speak, I'll vomit over us both. I manage a nod.

He leads me a short distance away. I can still see the spot of my attack, but I feel safer further from it. Although the risk of me vomiting remains pretty high, my breathing returns to normal and I start to calm down. Feeling more secure, I'm able to continue the story of that night. I can't seem to stop. And whereas before I'd often avoided saying certain phrases or softened some details to make it easier for Paddy to hear, a relentless and torrential downpour of words now cascade from my lips with unfiltered ferocity.

―――――――――――― " " ――――――――――――

PADDY

I've read her right. Her cheeks may still be white, but with the sounds and sights of the builders receding, she appears calmer now, able to return to the retelling of that night. Her words gather as she forces the memories from her in the very place where they were first formed.

―――――――――――― " " ――――――――――――

ANNA

A well-dressed lady walks in front of me as I'm describing some less-than-pleasant details and I'm struck by embarrassment. I don't want her to think badly of me, but I can't stop recounting the story. It's as though the restraints that have bound my speech for twenty years have suddenly been severed. I direct a certain amount of envy at this chic stranger. I wonder if she's on a lunch break, going back to her perfect job. And while I love the life I have created, there's a part of me that wishes I was her, living her seemingly trauma-free life. I want to chase after her and tell her that I've been happily married for thirteen years, I'm a good mother, I have two degrees, a dog, a house, a car, all the trappings of societal success. I also want to tell her that I love her Louboutins.

As I look longingly after the stylish lady and her beautiful, red-lacquered soles, I become more aware of my surroundings – the traffic, Paddy, the birds. I'm reminded of the sparrow I heard this morning and it soothes me even more. As I look around, I'm struck by how young everyone looks. Whenever I have pictured this place, in nightmares or flashbacks, I'm eighteen years old, but being here makes it very obvious that I'm not. The fashionable lady has reminded me of my age, and it helps me to differentiate between then and now.

---------------- " " ----------------

PADDY

Anna stops talking, the account finally out. She's added nothing to my understanding of what happened, yet hearing her describe her experience here feels hugely significant.

She has come to this tiny spot in the middle of the city, to a place that's haunted her for decades. And she's not been silenced or forced to detach by dissociating or had her breath completely stolen by a panic attack.

It's a little scruffy patch of grass in front of a church, yet in Anna's head it had acquired the power of a black and boiling sea.

A church. There's a sharp and familiar stab of anger in my chest at what happened here, in full view of this building. Another violation, I cannot help thinking, that was overlooked. Ignored.

I push my thoughts aside to focus on Anna.

And what I see gives me hope. She has come here and spoken and the waves have not swallowed her whole. She has beaten the tempest.

ANNA

Paddy and I walk a little further away and sit together on a wall. We are both silent for a moment. I haven't dissociated, had a long-lasting public panic attack, vomited, cried or had to face any of the other fears I'd had prior to this trip. I feel a little numb, empty perhaps, and unable to quite access what I feel.

'How are you doing?' he asks.

'I don't know. Everything seems a bit... boring?' I search my brain for a better word. 'Undramatic, maybe?'

'I don't think that's a bad thing, at all,' he offers.

I swing my legs against the wall. In contrast to how I felt this morning, I genuinely feel OK. And, of course, he's right, 'undramatic' isn't a bad thing. It's the very thing that my life needs right now.

We're sitting with our backs to the site of my trauma and it seems symbolic – as if the past is finally behind me. I've looked into the depths of the abyss, faced the spectre of my fears, and I have survived.

CHAPTER 32

'The wound is the place where light enters you.'
RUMI

PADDY

After our trip, when I hoped that Anna was edging towards a calmer, more-settled place, I realised that I was heading in the opposite direction.

During the time we had worked together, life had gradually changed. Together with my wife, I was caring for two teenage daughters, one with special needs. I was also tending to the increasing needs of my elderly parents, who were at that point in their late eighties. Demands on my time were piling up and I was often stressed and overwhelmed.

The phrase 'wounded healer', now a popular, much-used term within therapy, partly describes the state I was in, practising as a counsellor while feeling less than optimal. First coined by Jung, it originally expressed the idea that analysts, therapists and physicians are driven to treat others' pain because they themselves have experienced it in the past. As Jung put it, 'it is his own hurt that gives a measure of his power to heal'. The most obvious example of the wounded healer is Viktor Frankl, who survived four years in Nazi concentration camps and went on to become an influential psychiatrist (and the author of *Man's Search for Meaning*). In addition, the term acknowledges that a physician's pain can be both motivation and impediment (think of Hugh Laurie's character in the television series *House*), the idea being that if unexamined or unresolved, pain can result in destructive or contaminating behaviour.

Today, the term appears to have a broader application and also refers to the understanding that therapists will experience periods of poor mental health. They are human, after all, subject to the same problems and traumas as anyone else. At the same time, like others in the caring profession, they have an obligation to examine and process their pain, so that it can be a force for good (or if that's not possible, at least contained) in the counselling room.

Slowly, I came to realise that this very process was necessary for me. Without closer examination, there was a danger my troubles would leak into the counselling space.

The issues were easy enough to forget by day, when I functioned well enough. After dark, however, I began to unravel. Some nights I fell asleep only to wake in the small hours and lie, my body tensed, my mind whirring away, until dawn. Other nights, I got no sleep at all.

I knew that my nocturnal wrestling went beyond anxieties

about my caring duties which, while persistent, were straightforward enough. I sensed that what lay beneath was something more complicated.

When I thought about Ampleforth, and specifically about the revelations of sexual abuse, I felt as if I was on an emotional see-saw.

I veered between outrage – a deep anger with the monastic community and all those who'd covered up its crimes, one so intense that I fantasised about taking a wrecking ball to the school and monastery – and denial, where a soft veil fell across the darkness in my mind.

I was tired of this oscillation. I wanted to feel the ground beneath my feet. But to get off, I needed to understand what kept me in this in-between place.

I had snatches of therapy with Sue, tacked on to my monthly supervision, but the ghosts of my clients were always in the room, clouding that space. I realised that I needed some dedicated time with another counsellor, in which I could focus on myself, free from my clients' personalities and narratives.

Given my early experience with Jungian psychoanalysis, it might have made sense to seek a more human encounter. But I had met enough of them by now to know that not all Jungians are aloof. Besides, for all its faults, analysis in my twenties had been a rigorous experience, one that had dived deep into my unconscious and delivered lasting results. I needed it again now. To look at my inner world as uncompromisingly as Anna had hers.

I found a therapist called Jonathan whose profile appealed to me. He had a kind face (always helps), extensive training and an understanding of children with special needs. During our first session, he came across as warm and accepting, curious about my dreams and a man who was unafraid to maintain silence if he felt it might be of value. From the get-go, I liked him and the way he worked.

For the next six months, in between speaking about parenting and my parents, I discussed the confusing, contradictory feelings I had about Ampleforth. Slowly, an explanation for them came to light.

Denial could be triggered by the most inconsequential encounter – a throwaway conversation or small talk at a party – but always with the same kind of person: middle class, obsessed with education. They'd hear my accent, detect a whiff of public school and, eventually, ask where I had gone. I'd say 'Ampleforth' and they'd almost purr with pleasure.

The typical responses were: 'My cousin/brother/best friend went there.' Or: 'Wasn't Rupert Everett/James Norton at Ampleforth?'

(The school is very proprietorial about its old boys, particularly the famous ones, parading high achievers in the journal it publishes every year, as if Ampleforth alone is responsible for their adult triumphs. Ironically, Everett has described his time there as 'a heart-breaking experience that you never quite recover from', while Norton said in an interview that he needed therapy to get over his experience of being bullied at the school.)

As I discovered through these conversations, many people still regard Ampleforth as the Catholic Eton. Despite all the horrors revealed in page after page of the IICSA report, for them, it remains an alluring bastion of prestige.

More surprising to me, old boys, as that glitzy party I attended had proved, could be equally in its thrall. Every now and then, I'd meet a middle-aged alumnus who still loved to attend school reunions or to travel up to Yorkshire for Mass in the abbey church. Some of them had even sent their children there.

Time and again, when I'd encountered these people, I softened and slipped into a more comfortable place. I was back in the club, no longer angry. Ampleforth – a school with such a cult following – couldn't possibly be a place of darkness. At times, I felt like what I'd read in the report, the unease I'd sensed in the air as a student, were fictions.

In pinning down in therapy the effect of these encounters, I was able to understand why the swings occurred. And in discussing the IICSA report, I felt their impact less, because Jonathan shared my horror and validated my truth. I was finally standing on more solid ground.

I also told him about the apprehension I felt at school. I realised that the time I spent boarding from the age of seven to seventeen was in a state of hypervigilance. At Ampleforth, where there was a near-constant sense of danger, it was dialled right up.

The school hummed with a malevolent energy and barbaric flashes of violence were the norm. One evening in my boarding house, I was snatched, dragged into the nearest toilet cubicle and forced onto my knees. As the sharp tang of urine filled my nostrils, my head was plunged into the bowl. Then, the flush was pulled, icy water drenching my hair and filling the bowl, while a hand was pressed firmly to the back of my head to keep me under. When my lungs were close to bursting, I was hauled out, gasping, as two older boys standing behind me convulsed with laughter. I had been bog-washed, just like that human rights lawyer at his public school. Torture for fun, for the sheer hell of it.

One Saturday afternoon when I was about thirteen, I returned to my dormitory to a scene I will never forget. A boy in the third year – a quiet, unassuming teen – had been stripped naked by his peers and tied to the four corners of the entrance to his cubicle with dressing gown cords. He was spread-eagled like Leonardo da Vinci's *Vitruvian Man*, utterly exposed and vulnerable, his genitalia covered in shaving foam. The boys responsible were standing around laughing and joshing. One of them held up a pornographic magazine, forcing the naked boy to look. When this terrified but hormonal teen showed signs of sexual arousal, they screamed with delight and disgust. It was an act of extraordinary cruelty that was expertly designed to elicit total humiliation, and it left me in a state of shock and terror for weeks. If they could do this to a boy their own age, what did they have in store for someone in the first year?

Predatory sexual behaviour was standard, with younger students openly objectified and pursued by older pupils.

Boys as young as thirteen would be invited to sixth-formers' rooms for coffee, tea and a cigarette (sixth-formers could smoke with their parents' permission – lighting up in spaces where the walls were hung with Indian drapes and tie-dyed sheets, tinderbox conditions that miraculously never resulted in a fire). The 'pretty boys', as they were known, would be ogled and touched, intimately if sixth-formers got the chance. In such a cold, inhumane environment, it was all too easy to succumb to the attention, but there was nothing balanced and consensual about this activity. A sixth-former who briefly became obsessed with me visited the dormitory late at night and tried to put his hand under my duvet but was disturbed at the last minute by my patrolling housemaster. When I hit puberty, I felt that kind of attraction myself and made it clear to one younger boy that I fancied him. Not long after leaving, I returned to the school and apologised to him for any discomfort I had made him feel, but for years my actions left me with a sense of shame and collusion. I had become part of the problem, part of the same oppressive cycle.

It wasn't just the boys who made you feel unsafe. The monks also had an unsettling effect. It wasn't something that you could put your finger on, but thinking of them now, floating silently into the abbey church on Sunday in black robes, hoods pulled over their heads, I'm reminded of the Dementors in *Harry Potter*. Silent, dark, sinister.

These were the things I could see. There was also the unseen.

I did not personally experience sexual abuse and I had no knowledge of any instances beyond a few rumours. But Jonathan helped me to understand how the widespread but indiscernible nature of abuse inevitably contaminated the institution, poisoning the very air the students breathed.

It's impossible to know how the school environment affected individuals in the long term, but I know what it did to me.

As a therapist, I've learned that sensitive, porous clients often feel the unspoken. This can be a piece of inherited generational trauma or a partner or close relative projecting a feeling they themselves cannot fully articulate. I think the emotion I absorbed at that school – where boys' lives were being destroyed and the very worst of crimes were covered up – was guilt.

This will sound very Catholic, but I believe it led to a drive for penance. As an adult, I had often felt responsible for upsets or rifts that had nothing to do with me. On the positive side, this trait fed into my career as a therapist, fuelling a desire to bring peace to my clients. On the negative, however, I had at times felt like I was a destroyer, obligated to soothe and repair people for the rest of my life.

Therapy with Jonathan taught me two very simple but incredibly powerful truths.

I had not wrought the destruction that occurred at my school.

It was not my guilt.

It took me to the age of fifty-four to make those connections

– sometimes that's just how it is – but establishing them felt profound and liberating.

Yet, despite the shift in me, there remained a tiny worm of doubt and I became convinced that the only way to truly consolidate my learning was to make a journey, just like the one Anna had embarked on.

CHAPTER 33

'Surviving is important. Thriving is elegant.'
Maya Angelou

ANNA

In the days following our trip to Bristol, I continued to feel indifferent, perhaps even numb. Like I was standing at the edge of a perfectly still lake where ripples barely disturb the surface.

'How have you been since Bristol?' Paddy asked during our next session.

'I'm OK. I keep waiting to have a night terror, a flashback, an outburst of emotion, but there's been nothing. So far.' As I sat in front of Paddy, I felt calm for the very first time. Stronger, even. My body wasn't fidgeting, my breathing was calm and slow. And I was no longer perched on the furthest end of the sofa away from him.

'And can I ask – self-harming?'

'None. I can't even remember the last time.'

'Perhaps it's still percolating through?' he offered.

'I don't know. It's been over a week. I think I would have had something by now?'

'This is new territory for me, but I hope so.'

And as the weeks passed, I began to notice that things which previously would have triggered a flashback or a panic attack, such as a belt or a necklace, became normal everyday objects. I didn't like them and I was aware of their meanings, but I could view them neutrally rather than as something visceral and traumatic.

" "

PADDY

A therapeutic relationship typically ends in one of three ways – the client sends a message to say they're finished, they simply fail to show up or there's a conversation prompted by either the client or counsellor which shapes the ending in a more mutually satisfactory way.

If it's me starting that conversation, it's usually in one of two circumstances. The first is if the client is vacillating, procrastinating or resisting, for whatever reason, in fully engaging with their issues. In this instance, talking about an ending can be useful. With luck, the client acknowledges the stagnation and becomes motivated. Even sensing that time is limited can be hugely motivating. Like a stick of dynamite thrown on the hardest of grounds, it breaks the surface and allows for excavation. Clients may also begin to consider other therapeutic routes better suited to their personality. I'm more than happy to help them. After all, it's not the vehicle but the destination that counts. Some of the more pragmatic, logical clients – the ones who want measurable, structured sessions and feel less enthusiastic about examining their distant past or the contents of their dreams – often opt for a counsellor who offers CBT at this juncture. CBT is usually a time-limited approach that looks at the here and now, providing specific exercises to build coping mechanisms or challenge unhelpful thoughts.

The other circumstance is when there's a feeling in the room, often shared by both counsellor and client, that the work is nearing completion.

Coming from the counsellor, that conversation can sometimes prompt difficult feelings in the client, often around loss, separation or abandonment, even if they're ready to end the sessions. Talking about endings is an opportunity to discuss those emotions, as well as their therapy experience in general. This is a chance to reinforce what they have learned and identify and tackle anything that still needs to be achieved. To look at what might happen in the future and what the relationship has been like for them.

It was Anna who first mentioned finishing.

———————————— " " ————————————

ANNA

'I can see the end of counselling,' I said, some weeks after our trip.

Paddy said nothing, but the smile on his face invited me to say more.

'I haven't had any nightmares or flashbacks since Bristol and I haven't self-harmed in months. In fact, it hasn't even crossed my mind,' I said, amazed to hear those words out loud.

'This is wonderful to hear, Anna,' Paddy said, his smile broadening.

Lola stretched on the floor and let a long, satisfied sigh escape her mouth, making us both laugh.

'Stopping self-harming was your specific goal for so long. But it appears to have simply ceased to become necessary, because you've processed your trauma.'

I nodded. 'I think so.' There was more. 'I'm also feeling increasingly confident. I find myself sharing my story with others. In fact, I don't seem to be able to keep my mouth shut.'

'This from a client who didn't want to speak at the start.'

'That's true. I also think this is the first time I haven't dreaded seeing you – no offence, but I've hated coming here every week.'

'None taken,' he said, smiling again. 'You've done incredibly well. Do you remember our first session? How you turned up at a strange man's house in the middle of nowhere? The pain of that hornet sting. Me arriving late. Not a promising start, was it?'

'It really wasn't.'

'You were always perched on the edge of the sofa during those early sessions, ready to bolt.'

'I wanted to run so many times.'

'But you stayed.'

We sat in quiet contemplation before Paddy spoke again.

'Can I ask, why me, a male counsellor?'

'I didn't think about you being a man or that I'd have to tell you my deepest, darkest secrets. Most of my doctors were male, including my gynaecologist. I thought counselling was just an extension of the medical profession.'

'You thought I'd be able to fix you?'

'Exactly. When I first came, I was suffering from panic attacks and nightmares. I knew I was broken and hoped you'd cure me – without having to uncover what I was in denial about. Or what I'd been repressing.'

'You weren't broken, Anna.'

'I know that now,' I added quietly. 'I thought I'd been successfully compartmentalising all these years. I had a great marriage, three children, two degrees and was able to hold down a successful job. But eventually, I realised I'd been repressing everything.'

'Even when you were having flashbacks, sleeping one hour a night – for months – you were still highly functional.'

'Yes – I felt like a swan at times. Calm and serene above the surface, but frantically kicking under the water to keep myself afloat.'

'You were so resilient.'

" "

PADDY

In our effort to recognise and bear witness to a client's pain, we sometimes run the risk of not validating their resilience. We're too eager to get them to examine their wounds and we fail to acknowledge how well they are coping, mistaking resilience for avoidance.

The type of resilience that helps us live and function is one I'm very familiar with. Boarding school pupils are forced to adapt to being away from home at an early age, to existing without their family, the comforts of home life, the food they are familiar with and the bed they enjoy sleeping in. In adapting to the deprivations of school life – to what was, at least pre-2000, a very basic existence of communal living in draughty old buildings – they acquire some skills. Former boarders are often quick to adjust to life at university, to careers that require travel and time away from home, and also to physical discomfort. This is not always a bad thing. Sometimes, we all need to cope with being away from our loved ones, to adjust to living with strangers or without our creature comforts. It's when it crosses the line into repression – when we ignore the wounds of our past and how they're affecting us in the present – that it becomes problematic.

At first, Anna demonstrated the kind of resilience that allowed her to cope. She'd forged a life despite the horrors of her past, gained two degrees, built a career, brought up three children. These were admirable achievements. But Anna also recognised that mentally, the past was pushing at a door and her coping mechanism was beginning to fray at the edges.

Within therapy, however, she found a deeper and more meaningful version of resilience. At times, she felt overwhelmed by the process of revealing and examining her past, week after week. So often, Anna wanted to end counselling and retreat to a safer place of suppression or denial. But instead, she returned, navigating her sessions with increased strength and perseverance.

She felt all the pain and pushed through anyway. And as a result, Anna built her resilience on a bedrock of granite.

———————————— " " ————————————

ANNA

Therapy had gifted me with a new-found sense of freedom and I began to wonder what my future would bring. I'd been privileged to spend the past few years at home with my three children, but they were now all in pre-school or school. I had an MSc and a solid career as an engineering consultant. It was stable and respected, yet I had always felt unfulfilled.

I was profoundly changed by my time in therapy and I began to reassess what success and contentment really meant to me. Paddy had shown me how powerful and transformative connections could be.

So, with Sam's encouragement, I began another journey: a quest to become a counsellor myself, during which I made a promise to always wear interesting shoes, for the clients that wouldn't, or couldn't, make eye contact.

CHAPTER 34

PADDY

For months, I veered between thinking that a visit to Ampleforth was a great idea – the only way to finally bring about a permanent shift – and a totally unnecessary expedition. I had done the work and didn't feel any significant discomfort. What was the point?

It was late summer and I was driving north to stay with an old friend in Northumberland. At the time, I convinced myself that I had no intention of visiting the school, but looking back now, I wonder whether my unconscious was at the wheel.

I had planned to break the journey in a village in North Yorkshire called Scampston, where there was a garden open to the public. As I headed east from the A1, signs began to appear for a slew of villages. In an instant, the names transported me back to my teenage years, making my stomach churn and my head spin. Kilburn, Coxwold, Stonegrave, Oswaldkirk. Finally, Ampleforth itself.

I made it to the garden, determined to be distracted. I also decided to plot another route back to the motorway, so I avoided encountering any more reminders of my school days.

It was raining lightly. The garden was all but deserted. There were a few hardcore visitors in kagools wandering the lawns and pathways.

I picked up a leaflet and read about the place's history. An old walled garden of vegetable beds had been transformed by a famous contemporary designer into 'rooms' of planting, each with their own distinct mood. There were architectural swaying grasses that drew the eye across a wide vista. Mixed beds filled with a variety of colours and shapes compelled me to stoop to study flower heads, stems and leaves. In another room, a small pyramid invited me to climb. Standing at its peak, the view through the drizzle spanned over the tops of cherry trees and a meadow of wild flowers. Each room was distinct yet part of a harmonious whole. I felt calm.

Back in the car, that serenity began to disintegrate as I studied a map on my phone. Avoiding Ampleforth required what looked like a slow, torturous route across the Yorkshire Moors, adding more than an hour to my journey time. I decided to head back the way I'd come, relying on a set of emotional blinkers that would inure me to all the signage that seemed to point in only one direction.

I followed the satnav. There was absolutely no reason to go anywhere near Ampleforth, which sat on a minor B road that led nowhere useful.

I think at some point I must have stopped looking at the satnav, because suddenly, I was on what we Ampleforth students used to call the Top Road, the route directly above the campus.

My stomach twisted, just as it had when I was a teenager in my parents' car, as they drove me back to school at the beginning of term.

I had a choice: I could drive away. Or I could do the thing that some part of me had perhaps known for weeks or even longer was necessary. That some part of me had even engineered all along.

A spark of resolve ignited in my chest. I thought of Anna in Bristol, of the moment she realised she was no longer an eighteen-year-old student but a grown woman with children. Like the city, she'd moved on. In the same way, I wasn't a schoolboy any more, not small and insignificant, but an adult.

I took a right turn down past the rear of the abbey church and the monastery before emerging in front of the entire campus. Now, I was on a road that would lead me into the heart of the school.

Up ahead was a wooden fence blocking my passage. A gate in front of it was locked, a CCTV camera perched on a post. When I was a student, the school and monastery belonged to the same fluid campus, where monks mingled freely with the boys in their roles as housemasters, teachers and officers in the cadet force – with catastrophic, life-destroying consequences. Now, the school was sealed off from the monastic community, a sign of the clear division Ofsted had recommended to protect the students from abuse.

Turning around, I noticed a sign by the abbey that declared the church open to the public. 'All are welcome,' it said. I stared at the words in disbelief. The monastic community – the source of all the pain and suffering inflicted on so many boys over decades – was still at large.

I didn't really believe that a member of the public who happened to wander into the abbey was immediately at risk of sexual abuse, or that every member of the community was a danger, but it felt ludicrous and insulting to infer that this was a place of safety and sanctuary for all.

The spark in my chest became a flame.

Driving down the valley, I parked by a cricket pavilion.

Looking back, I took in the view. It was a scene I'd revisited in my head hundreds, possibly thousands, of times in the decades since leaving.

Jonathan and I had discussed how I might 'respond' to Ampleforth if I ever visited. Could I step out onto the pristine flat grass of the cricket pitch and piss on the crease? Or drop my trousers and take a shit?

Term was over, yet I felt a hundred eyes on me from the windows overlooking the valley.

I managed to piss against the pavilion but only felt the relief of emptying my bladder. Not the statement of disgust I'd hoped for.

My heart was still beating furiously, but something inside me was shifting.

Anna had cemented Bristol in her mind as a place of demons and darkness. Returning there had shown her a city that was living and breathing. With Ampleforth, it wasn't so straightforward. But I was beginning to see it with a fresh perspective.

Sitting at the head of a gently sloping valley, Ampleforth has one of the most beautiful settings of any school. At the heart of the site is the abbey church, designed by Sir Giles Gilbert Scott, the architect responsible for Battersea Power Station, Bankside Power Station (now Tate Modern) and Liverpool's Anglican Cathedral. Like those buildings, it has a powerful, almost industrial feel, although its box-like forms are tempered with a hint of ecclesiastical Gothic in the details. On Sundays, the abbey's bells would peal before Mass, a deep, resonant sound that echoed across the landscape. Elsewhere, buildings reflect the style of the time in which they were constructed: art deco curves, the brightly coloured detailing of postmodernism, the soft organic shapes of contemporary architecture.

It was undoubtedly built to impress. To create a sense of awe. To seduce.

In Bristol, Anna could confidently piece together the events of her trauma by visiting the places where her ordeals had occurred. After all those years, after all the comments that dismissed or denied her experience, she knew, in her chest and stomach, that her trauma was real, that events had unfolded just as she'd described them to me in sessions. She could trust her memories, so often undermined by others. It had not been an easy moment. Anna was then assailed by the clarity of her understanding, that horrific things had indeed happened. But it was the start of a powerful healing process, as the sites of her nightmares were slowly robbed of their power in daylight.

In the same way, the unease I'd felt all those years before, which eventually found a shape when I read the IICSA report, sharpened in that moment.

Ampleforth could throw all of its natural beauty at me, all of its impressive architecture. But it could not deny the truth.

It felt like a powerful voice was speaking directly into my ear: 'Bad things did happen in this place.'

It was enough. I climbed back into my car and drove away.

But as I headed north, doubts crept in. Compared to our trip to Bristol, where Anna and I lingered for about four hours, I had stayed at Ampleforth for no more than forty minutes.

Would it really be sufficient? Would it bring about the permanent shift I craved?

In Northumberland, I stayed with Frank, an old friend from school.

That evening, I sat down for dinner with him, his wife and their son and daughter, both of whom had recently studied at Ampleforth.

Frank is one of those old boys who appears blind to the scale of the school's crimes, despite them being well documented. Yet I have never questioned his decision to send his children there. The way I see it, it's none of my business and besides, there's no easy way to start a conversation about systemic sexual abuse.

His children are delightful – confident, kind, thoughtful and funny. Over dinner, they spoke animatedly about their time at the school. From their anecdotes, I was relieved to hear it emerge as a place of warmth and care, where they'd had a happy experience.

Before long, Frank and I joined in, sharing stories about our time there and laughing about memorable peers and eccentric teachers.

In bed that night, rather than experiencing the familiar pendulum swing that normally followed such a conversation, I saw only a set of balanced scales.

Before therapy and my visit to the school that day, any antipathy I might have harboured towards Ampleforth would have begun to unravel at this point. Frank's kids were well adjusted and joyous. There was an undeniable lightness about them. How could Ampleforth possibly be harmful or dangerous?

But all I experienced was certainty. I had my truth, and they had theirs – and the two truths could co-exist at the same time, without invalidating one another. As their stories and demeanour made clear, a positive student experience at the school is possible.

I saw too that my time there wasn't wall-to-wall darkness. There were many moments of light – the friendships that were formed, some of which have lasted a lifetime; the sense of humour we boys shared, which delivered many a belly laugh; the art room, where I learned how to draw under the guidance of a wonderful sculptor.

Staring at the ceiling, I thought about Frank, who remains a loyal supporter of a school that let so many of our peers down in the worst possible way. Why is that?

When I'd spoken to the old Amplefordian psychologist Jock at that party, he'd suggested that people's need to maintain a positive self-concept might explain their defence of the school. Jock talked about old boys simply refusing to accept that they're the type of person who would ever attend, or send their children to, a school where *that* kind of thing goes on. It made sense. But I wondered whether something else was also at play.

Children educated in the British boarding school system are torn from home and the love of their parents aged eight or, if they're lucky, thirteen. Either way, that moment can be devastating; as their mother and father drive away, the child is left with a deep sense of abandonment. They no longer feel safe. Their new home is a place of bewildering traditions and rules where even today, despite improved safeguarding practices, bullying and sexual abuse still occur (a fact sadly confirmed by Dino Nocivelli, a partner at Leigh Day, a law firm which specialises in representing survivors of childhood sexual abuse). If pupils feel scared, they can no longer go to their parents for a hug. Homesickness, a wholly inadequate word for the raw grief of separation, may follow. In *Boarding School Syndrome*, Jungian psychoanalyst Joy Schaverien's seminal book on the trauma caused by boarding, she writes:

'The profound anguish of the separation is actually bereavement, but it is not treated as such. Therefore the appropriate reaction, which would be acknowledgement and mourning, cannot take place.'

Many boarders quickly learn that sadness is frowned upon, in some cases even dangerous, so in time they shut down, effectively cauterising their emotions. Schaverien describes Theo, who realised at boarding school that 'to survive in an alien environment, there was little choice but to do violence to the tender self, to kill off the feeling state, in order to comply with the institution'. For some boarders, it's a way of being that can last a lifetime, resulting in broken relationships and addictive behaviours.

Lying in bed, an idea began to take shape in my head. Having been so brutally wrenched from the love and security of their parents, did some boarders find themselves forming fresh attachments, most likely at an unconscious level, to the 'new parent' – the boarding school. It's another possible explanation for why, in the face of such overwhelming evidence of systemic physical and sexual abuse, many old Amplefordians remain so fiercely loyal to, and supportive of, the school, even sending their children to be educated there. It is an act of fierce denial, but given their experience, who can blame them?

That night, something within me settled. I didn't need to cling to a binary rock, where all I had was hateful, destructive thoughts. I had my truth and now that allowed room for nuance and for others to have their truths.

I was certain of something else too. I could not have reached that sophisticated place of understanding – one that has since brought lasting peace – had my path not crossed with Anna's.

In scrutinising her past so unflinchingly, looking in the darkest of places, she showed me how to find light.

CHAPTER 35

'Though there are many phrases for the therapeutic relationship (patient/therapist, client/counselor, analysand/analyst, client/facilitator ... none of these phrases accurately convey my sense of the therapeutic relationship. Instead I prefer to think of my patients and myself as fellow travelers.'
IRVIN YALOM, THE GIFT OF THERAPY: AN OPEN LETTER TO A NEW GENERATION OF THERAPISTS AND THEIR PATIENTS

ANNA

I arrived a few minutes early, a barista greeting me. 'Table for one?'

'Erm, two actually.' I looked around the cafe, feeling slightly panicked. With the exception of our trip, Paddy and I were used to speaking in an atmosphere of near silence. This place was packed, voices clashing with the clatter of cutlery and china.

'Do you have any seats that are a bit quieter?' I asked, peering around the barista to look further into the back of the coffee shop. 'Preferably near a plug, if possible?' I patted my laptop case, as I planned to study when Paddy had gone.

I followed her to a booth in the back, and apart from three men in suits having what looked like a business meeting with their laptops and papers covering a small table, and two elderly ladies having coffee, it was quiet.

I pulled out a book and waited. A short while later, he arrived.

'Sorry I'm late, I couldn't find a space to park. Have you ordered? Nice to see you.' Paddy's words tumbled out.

'It's fine, don't worry. It's good to see you too.' This was a change in our familiar dynamic, it was now my turn to establish a calm atmosphere.

'How are you? It's been, what, over a year?' He sat, looking at the menu.

'Yes, it's been a while. I'm good, thank you.'

We ordered coffee and made small talk while we waited for our order to arrive.

'How's the training going?'

I was about to answer when the waitress approached with our drinks. I moved the book on the table – a crime novel co-written by Louise Voss and Mark Edwards – to make space.

Paddy tilted his head to read the title. 'Good?' he asked.

'Great. They write really well together.' I smiled.

We thanked the waitress and I waited for her to leave before continuing. 'In my email, I mentioned how I wanted to write about the Bristol trip?'

'Of course,' he said, adding sugar to his flat white and stirring.

―――――――――――― " " ――――――――――――

PADDY

After the trip, Anna and I had discussed contacting the researcher again. By now, Anna's enthusiasm had waned. She still felt compelled to help others through her experience but was more interested in writing a personal narrative than becoming a case study, which felt somehow dehumanising.

To me, narrative is a huge part of therapy. Clients come to their early sessions with what feels like the first draft of their story. It's thin, lacking in depth and seen from a single perspective. Over time, they build a fuller, richer account, one that allows them to see their life with more subtlety and perspective, so Anna didn't need to persuade me of its benefits.

As for what Anna had planned, I was convinced that her account would be compelling and moving. At the start of her therapy journey, emails had proved an additional medium for her to clarify or add texture to what she'd struggled to say in person. Terrified and sometimes mute in sessions, she came alive in those messages, her words full of rich description and metaphor, the turmoil of her inner world powerfully expressed and tangible on the page.

When she reached out, asking if I might meet for coffee to discuss writing about the trip, I assumed she wanted to talk about her own account. As it turned out, she had another idea.

--- " " ---

ANNA

'Sorry, I didn't answer your earlier question – training is going well, thank you. And actually, that brings me conveniently to the reason I asked you here. Since I've been studying to be a therapist, I keep returning to thoughts of how it was for you on that day. What was it like to literally walk in my footsteps around the city?' I took a sip of my Americano, burning my lip. 'I still want to write about it and I guess I was wondering how you'd feel about a collaboration?'

I paused, giving Paddy a chance to let the idea sink in.

'Hmm,' he said.

I heard the caution in his voice, noticed the subtle signs of discomfort in his body language, but pressed on. 'From what I can see, there are, sadly, lots of stories like mine, of men and women suffering and healing from trauma. There are also many books about therapy. What there doesn't seem to be is anything with a dual perspective.' I nodded towards the book on the table. 'Anything co-written.'

'That's a valid point,' he said, but he still sounded wary. 'The thing is, Anna, I'm convinced your story is powerful. You've gone from being a client who could barely speak to a therapist in training, one who aims to help others find their voices. It's undoubtedly inspirational. But it's your story and it should be heard in its entirety and without interruption. Does it need an additional voice, least of all a man's?'

I smiled, but it was not the answer I was looking for from him.

'Perhaps you can think about it?'

'Even if in the end, we agree to disagree?' he said.

'Of course.'

We moved on, chatting about my training, Paddy curious about what was current in therapeutic learning and joking about how out of practice he felt in my company as I discussed the texts I was reading.

———————— " " ————————

PADDY

The following morning, I emailed a friend who had, until recently, worked in publishing. To my surprise, she confirmed Anna's point. The market was indeed saturated with books about trauma written by both women and men. To stand a chance of gaining any traction, another book needed something to differentiate it from its competitors.

I emailed back, asking if an additional perspective, that of a therapist, for example, might work. She responded enthusiastically: 'That sounds intriguing.'

Niggling doubts still remained.

Was it too early? Anna was in a good place, would writing her story be retraumatising? Would the notoriously tough world of publishing – in which rejection from literary agents and publishers is par for the course – prove crushing to Anna's hard-won self-esteem?

Despite my doubts, I had to admit I was curious.

———————————— " " ————————————

ANNA

Weeks later, we met in the same coffee shop. The familiar barista greeted me warmly and showed me to a seat. Paddy arrived, looking less flustered this time.

As we ordered, he shared his thoughts and worries about the idea of collaborating. Although I heard and appreciated his concerns, I was adamant that I was in a good place and had been for a long time. The events seemed so distant and I was confident that I was resilient enough to withstand any rejections.

I told Paddy about the positive response I'd had from peers on my course whenever I spoke about our therapeutic relationship. 'They're fascinated. And, of course, they want to know about the trip we took, which was unusual, to say the least.'

'That's certainly true,' said Paddy.

It was still hard to gauge where he was on this.

'I'm sure people would be interested to hear what it was like for you to relive it with me that day.' I was on a roll. 'Not just then but throughout counselling. What is it like for a therapist to hear clients recall traumatic experiences?' I asked. 'And what's it like for a male counsellor to support a female client through her experience of rape?' I looked around, hoping that no one had heard me.

———————————— " " ————————————

PADDY

Thanks to the writings of Gabor Maté and Bessel van der Kolk, trauma as experienced by clients is much more widely understood now, but there's less out there about what it's like for a counsellor to hear clients recall their experiences. If I decided to work with Anna on this project, I had the opportunity to discuss the memories and emotions that her account of sexual violence brought to the surface for me. I could talk about my anger and how it proved to be a powerful therapeutic tool.

I felt a shift. I'd never shied away from self-disclosure if it helped Anna to open up. So she knew I'd been at boarding school. But now, no longer her therapist, it felt the right moment to tell Anna about my journey and how it might just work alongside hers in a book. Anna listened attentively, our roles reversed.

We left the cafe that day, agreeing to pick up the discussion again soon, and as we parted ways, I looked down. 'Nice shoes,' I said, pointing at Anna's pink Converse.

As I mulled over the idea, it struck me that while celebrated titles like *The Examined Life* by Stephen Grosz and Irvin Yalom's *Love's Executioner* have helped to illuminate therapeutic encounters from the counsellor's perspective, readers rarely hear from clients and how they experience the very same sessions. In writing with Anna, we had an opportunity to shine a light on the therapeutic process from both sides of the couch.

It was also a chance to show that therapists are not experts who have all the answers. At times, we both felt lost and frustrated and were searching for answers. In writing the book, I could examine what therapeutic interventions we tried – what worked and what didn't. I could look at the mistakes made and the lessons learned along the way and show how my fallibility proved key to Anna's healing.

―――――――――――― " " ――――――――――――

ANNA

I wanted to give Paddy ample time to process the idea I'd proposed. In order for it to work, we both needed to be fully invested in the decision to collaborate. I was sure that my story could help others who had suffered from sexual violence, but I also felt very strongly that the narrative would benefit from an additional voice. And given what Paddy had told me about the impact of our work on him, it struck me that even though we had shared the same voyage, it had shaped us in very different ways.

———————————— " " ————————————

PADDY

Anna had always been impatient for results in therapy and that same impatience must have reasserted itself as I weighed up my decision – a process that took weeks – although she was far too polite to say.

Even though Anna was no longer my client, I discussed the potential project with Sue to help me reach a conclusion. My supervisor helped me to consider the shift that writing would demand of Anna and me. It would mean moving from a relationship of former therapist and client to co-writers and collaborators. When examining it during supervision, I felt confident that sufficient time had elapsed for us to make a distinction between one dynamic and another. That was enough. I was in.

And so the process began, that table in the back of a cafe as important to us now as the counselling room had been in the past. Whereas before the background to our conversations had been birdsong or an occasional sigh from Lola, now our work was set against the bustle of that coffee shop. Waiters bursting from the kitchen swing doors to deliver steaming mugs or plates of food to the regulars in the booths and tables around us. The group of exhausted new mums, their sleeping babies in prams, who met mid-morning for coffee and cake. The bookworm who was always so lost in a novel that her cappuccino went cold. The elderly couple who ate matching plates of scrambled eggs and smoked salmon in companionable silence.

We had a new relationship, but Anna was still my former client and I couldn't help but worry about her occasionally. She was adamant that her therapeutic gains were well established and that she was robust enough to withstand what writing might bring. But what if the demands of the book – remembering in forensic detail, finding words to describe the murky distant past – dredged up old pain and reopened wounds?

As we structured the book and wrote some initial chapters, my concern lingered.

Until one day, I noticed that it had evaporated.

It wasn't easy for Anna to recall and shape her painful memories. During our sessions, she'd expressed a hope that one day, such an exercise would be as unemotional an experience as reading a shopping list. But in reality, the memories still had weight; the power to bring tears to her eyes. To mine as well. But the difference now was that once Anna had cried, she returned to solid ground, to a place of resilience, where the past was well integrated and no longer had the power to traumatise. Therapy really had worked.

Sometimes, writing and editing the accounts that covered my childhood, I cried about my experience. But the ease with which I connected to my emotions was a relief. I felt human again; my feelings were no longer stymied but flowing freely through me.

As with all stories, there was an arc to Anna's. As we wrote, and she encouraged me to view my life in the focused way that she had hers, I saw mine more clearly.

Narrative arcs are a device, a way of structuring a story to give the reader a sense of closure, when in reality, Anna and I have continued to live our lives, with all the attendant joys and challenges, long after the final page. But the resolution I felt in writing was profound, as satisfying as any I'd experienced after a rich period of learning in counselling.

In therapy, we sometimes experience resolution in a wordless way. We feel better, even if we can't quite articulate why, and that can be enough. This book has provided me with all the words and, on this occasion, they're comforting. There's a solidity to them.

With Anna, our best therapeutic work was achieved when we collaborated, when we remembered our shared humanity. A balance. It was also true of writing.

Then, as now, fellow travellers, in it together.

EPILOGUE

'We depend on the other in order for us to be fully who we are.'
Archbishop Desmond Tutu

ANNA

For the majority of my time in therapy, I just wanted my rapes not to have happened. I tried suppressing, ignoring, denying, reframing and arguing with my therapist. Anything to avoid acknowledging the fact that I had been raped. It was only when I accepted what had happened to me and began to process the events and work through all the painful emotions I'd repressed that I started to heal.

***

My daughter told me this morning that every seven years, all the cells in our bodies are replaced. This means that mine will have changed three times since X raped me. They've been completely replaced. But for the majority of the past two decades, I felt tainted. X didn't just touch me physically or sexually. He reached far beyond the corporeal, and it was his betrayal of my trust that completely broke my heart. And it felt like no amount of years or cell replacement would ever undo that. I felt damaged and broken.

When I eventually decided to find a counsellor, nearly twenty years later, I didn't know where to start. I would lie awake at night, my phone turned away from my husband and type 'counsellors within twenty miles' into the search engine, before deleting the words, too ashamed to be seeking help. Eventually, after making it on to a directory of counsellors, I was overwhelmed with therapists, all with letters after their names that meant very little to me, offering hundreds of different types of therapies. Using my instinct, I picked the three that looked the least terrifying, narrowing my search down to two female and one male counsellors, ensuring that none of them were too local or likely to have a connection to anyone in my life. I didn't think deeply about whether I'd prefer to see a man or a woman. I wanted to feel better but rapidly and with as little pain as possible.

To my annoyance, I quickly discovered that therapy wasn't about receiving advice and being fixed but working through the most painful times of my life and entrusting my innermost thoughts and feelings to a complete stranger.

Trusting again after being so badly wounded was often like tiptoeing through a field of shattered glass, each step cautious and measured. I was fearful of any wrong move, where even the slightest whisper of vulnerability would feel like a betrayal in waiting. And so, at times, I was defensive or resistant to the therapeutic relationship. But Paddy was persistent, which often left me irritated and exasperated. He worked hard to win my trust and his fierce compassion ultimately showed me how to be compassionate to myself.

Admittedly, the trip we made to Bristol was a risk, but it was one that we were both willing to take. And by visiting the place of my nightmares with Paddy, he was able to help me substantiate the narrative that I had so painstakingly built. He encouraged me to believe in myself and my own memories, rather than looking for external validation, and trust my own experiences and feelings. In this way, the hurt caused by one man was healed by another's kindness. And although it was hugely helpful to have the responses that I should have received over twenty years ago, I am now able to provide them for myself.

I wrote this book to offer hope to anyone suffering from trauma and to show that it's never too late to seek help. By inviting the reader into the therapy room, I want to demystify counselling, normalise the process and remove the shame that is sometimes associated with asking for help. I must acknowledge at this point that I am privileged to be able to afford private therapy and that I did not face some of the barriers that many people have to when seeking counselling. Due to long waiting lists or the cost of therapy, it can be inaccessible to many.

In a 2020 report, Dame Vera Baird, the then Victims' Commissioner for England and Wales, said that rape had effectively been decriminalised. I aim to demonstrate that in the likely absence of justice, closure is possible. At least, it was for me.

Healing is not a destination but a continuous voyage, which is made easier by the support of others along the way. With Paddy's encouragement and compassion, I found strength and solace, enabling me to overcome past wounds. Along the way, I came to a deep understanding that my healing hasn't been the absence of emotions but the mastery of them. And where I once stepped with hesitation, I now tread with purpose and a new-found sense of freedom, empowered by the journey we shared.

I remember feeling devastated in one session that X would always win when Paddy calmly responded, 'X is just one person. There are two of us.' And as much as I hate to admit it, he was right.

———————— " " ————————

PADDY

In the final days of my therapy with Philip, when I was convinced that there was nothing left to learn after four years in that stuffy Hampstead room, I took a dream to him to analyse. By now, I'd got the hang of his technique, but this one had completely foxed me.

It was very short and, on the surface, very simple: I was

travelling on the Circle Line, searching in vain for Poplar. Round and round I went, the station never appearing.

I knew London well at the time. Poplar was on the Docklands Light Railway, not the Circle Line, so why was I being such an idiot in my dream?

Philip wasn't one for humour. His brand of Jungian psychoanalysis was a serious, focused business. But I remember him cracking a rare smile that day, barely able to contain his glee at the swift interpretation and the light it shone on my psyche.

'Are you sure it's not "popular" you're searching for?' he said.

He knew me well. I felt the internal 'aha', that small puncture of tension when the right interpretation lands.

At Ampleforth, sensing the overt threat from older boys – their pent-up violence, their predatory sexuality – and possibly a less conspicuous threat from the monastic community, I'd found a way to defend myself. I realised I could make people laugh. And when they laughed, they were disarmed, less likely to attack.

Being funny also made me popular.

That defence mechanism lasted well into my twenties, long after the threat had receded. I was always cracking jokes, ridiculing myself, being the entertainer or court jester.

That dream, and Philip's interpretation, proved to be a profound moment in my therapy. There was silence in the room and in that instant, I understood that I had been perpetuating a shtick or habit that, ultimately, was not serving me well.

Being a comedian keeps people at a distance. Someone with such nervous energy, who's always seeking a punchline, is not a person you can easily get close to. Equally, in being that man, I was keeping others at bay. My guard was constantly up, which meant that I couldn't connect either.

That day, I left Philip's office in a reflective mood. Quieter, calmer.

A switch is rarely flicked in therapy and I didn't change overnight. But over the months that followed, the understanding I'd gained percolated through me. I began to understand that humour was not something I needed to reach for every single time I found myself in groups of people or indeed with individuals. It could be used judiciously or not at all, giving me a chance to speak more thoughtfully or intimately and provide a space for others to express themselves. I didn't need to lampoon myself, which only served to diminish me. I could allow a fuller version of myself, the one I'd worked so hard to nourish on the inside, to be revealed to others.

I believe that fullness is the ultimate goal of therapy.

At the beginning of counselling, many clients declare that their goal is to be happy, to which I always reply by gently steering them towards Eleanor Roosevelt's quote, 'Happiness is not a goal – it's a by-product of a life well lived.'

That wonderful line has always stuck with me. A life well lived is full of meaning and fulfilment and is our very best hope of finding contentment, which is much more robust than the heightened but unsustainable state of happiness. Contentment allows us to roll with the punches that are inevitably thrown at us, rather than being floored.

To find meaning and fulfilment, to be that richer version of ourselves, we need to understand who we are and where our true needs and motivations lie. Therapy allows us to look deeply into the mirror, to see beyond the layer we elect to show others, to the parts we keep hidden.

That process is not a one-off. As we get older, the past has a habit of tripping us up. We assume we've put it to bed, but our relationship with it is fluid. We meet and fall in love and the relationships we had with our parents can prove key to how well we attach to our partner. We have children, reminding us of how we ourselves were parented. We lose loved ones, a pain that has the power to reignite earlier losses.

Such moments can prompt a need to return to therapy, to look within again so we can find fresh answers.

Anna also helped me to do just that. Not only in the way she looked unflinchingly at her past, which was inspirational, but in the chemical reaction that occurred as we worked. How her experience at the hands of one man helped me to connect with how I felt about those men who'd inflicted pain at my school. Ultimately, that led me to Jonathan and the clarity I gained with him and when I returned to my school.

Working with Anna has also changed how I function as a therapist. I am aware, more than ever, of what is really at work in a successful therapeutic relationship. Far beyond the empathy, active listening, unconditional positive regard or the ingenuity of our interventions is a human encounter. And if therapists dare to be a little more human, I truly believe that transformative work can happen.

Today, more than six years since we first began working together, Anna and I are now fellow therapists. We refer clients to each other. And I am proud to call her my friend.

ACKNOWLEDGEMENTS

ANNA AND PADDY

Thank you, Erin Kelly, for your invaluable thoughts on our original proposal.

Laura Williams at Greene & Heaton, for taking our unusual book to your heart and for finding us a special home at Biteback.

Lisa Goodrum and Ella Boardman at Biteback, for editing with such sensitivity and understanding.

Lola, for canine empathy and unconditional positive regard.

Early readers Louise Beech, Madeleine Black and Sarah Hilary, for giving us pre-publication courage when we were terrified, to put it mildly.

ANNA

Thank you to my wonderful friends Sára, Sophie, Siân, Cat, Karolina, Suzie and Sarah. I'm deeply grateful for the dog walks, gym sessions, supply of writing snacks and the adventures we've shared.

Carole and Mike, forever my biggest supporters. I love you both dearly.

Sam, for being a fantastic dad to our children and for your love and encouragement. I wouldn't be who I am today without you.

And finally, a message to eighteen-year-old me: it gets better, I promise.

PADDY

Thank you, Jock Eldon, Dino Nocivelli and Alex Renton, for your expertise with my boarding school chapters.

Author friends Sarah Hilary, Ed James, Erin Kelly, Syd Moore and Olivia Isaac-Henry, for laughter, encouragement and mental-health maintenance.

Greta Stoddart, for next-level friendship.

Sue Prowse, for supervisory wisdom and insight.

Jonathan Wilkes, for therapy that brought lasting change.

The Prussia Cove library massive, for writerly solidarity and sporadic hush.

Vanessa Neuling, for love.